BLUEPRINTS
Q&A Step 3 Psychiatry

Second Edition

BLUEPRINTS
Q&A Step 3 Psychiatry

Second Edition

James Brian McLoone, MD, DFAPA
Chairman, Department of Psychiatry and
Director, Psychiatry Residency Training Program and Medical Student Clerkship
Banner Good Samaritan Medical Center
Clinical Professor of Psychiatry
University of Arizona College of Medicine—Phoenix Campus
Phoenix, Arizona

Series Editor:

Michael S. Clement, MD, FAAP
Mountain Park Health Center
Clinical Lecturer in Family and Community Medicine
University of Arizona College of Medicine
Consultant, Arizona Department of Health Services
Phoenix, Arizona

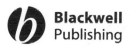

Blackwell
Publishing

Blackwell Publishing, Inc., 350 Main Street, Malden, Massachusetts 02148-5018, USA
Blackwell Publishing Ltd, 9600 Garsington Road, Oxford OX4 2DQ, UK
Blackwell Publishing Asia Pty Ltd, 550 Swanston Street, Carlton, Victoria 3053, Australia

04 05 06 07 5 4 3 2 1

ISBN: 1-4051-0397-3

Library of Congress Cataloging-in-Publication Data

Blueprints Q&A Step 3. Psychiatry / [edited by] James Brian McLoone.—2nd ed.
    p. ; cm.—(Blueprints Q&A Step 3)
    ISBN 1-4051-0397-3 (pbk.)
    1. Psychiatry—Examinations, questions, etc.   2. Physicians—Licenses—United
States—Examinations—Study guides.   I. McLoone, James Brian.   II. Title: Blueprints Q&A
Step 3.   III. Title: Psychiatry.   IV. Series: Blueprints. Q&A Step 3 series. [DNLM:
1. Psychiatry—Examination Questions. WM 18.2 B6582 2005]

    RC457.B582 2005
    616.89′0076—dc22

                                                                        2004013546

A catalogue record for this title is available from the British Library

Acquisitions: Nancy Anastasi Duffy
Development: Kate Heinle
Production: Jennifer Kowalewski
Cover design: Hannus Design Associates
Interior design: Mary McKeon
Typesetter: Techbooks in New Delhi, India
Printed and bound by Capital City Press in Berlin, VT

For further information on Blackwell Publishing, visit our website:
www.blackwellmedstudent.com

Notice: The indications and dosages of all drugs in this book have
been recommended in the medical literature and conform to the practices of
the general community. The medications described do not necessarily have
specific approval by the Food and Drug Administration for use in the
diseases and dosages for which they are recommended. The package insert for
each drug should be consulted for use and dosage as approved by the FDA.
Because standards for usage change, it is advisable to keep abreast of
revised recommendations, particularly those concerning new drugs.

The publisher's policy is to use permanent paper from mills that
operate a sustainable forestry policy, and which has been manufactured from
pulp processed using acid-free and elementary chlorine-free practices.
Furthermore, the publisher ensures that the text paper and cover board used
have met acceptable environmental accreditation standards.

Contents

Contributors

Elizabeth Baytion Munshi, MD
PGY-3 Psychiatry Resident
Banner Good Samaritan Medical Center
Phoenix, Arizona

Tracy L. Crews, MD
Chief Resident, Department of Psychiatry
Banner Good Samaritan Medical Center
Phoenix, Arizona

Derek Deibler, MD
PGY-3 Psychiatry Resident
Banner Good Samaritan Medical Center
Phoenix, Arizona

Adam R Koelsch, MD
Chief Resident, Department of Psychiatry
Banner Good Samaritan Medical Center
Phoenix, Arizona

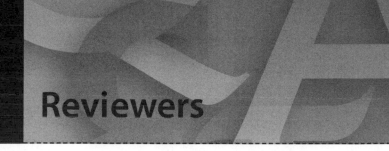

Reviewers

Elias Hsu, MD
Resident, Urology
Baylor College of Medicine
Houston, Texas

Christopher T. Starnes, MD
Senior Resident, Internal Medicine
University of South Carolina
Columbia, South Carolina
University of Virginia
Charlottesville, Virginia

Amber S. Podoll, MD
PGY-2 Resident, Medicine and Pediatrics
Baylor College of Medicine
Houston, Texas

Preface

Thank you! We know that you, our customers, have successfully used the first edition of the Blueprints Q&A series to study for Boards and shelf exams. We also learned that those of you in physician assistant, nurse practitioner, and osteopath programs have found the series helpful to review for Boards and rotation exams.

At Blackwell, we think of our customers as our secret weapon. For every book Blackwell publishes, we rely heavily on the opinions of our customers, and we credit much of our success to the feedback we get from you. Your comments, suggestions—even complaints—help determine everything from content to features to the design of our books. The second edition of the Blueprints Q&A series is an excellent example of how much influence your feedback truly has:

- You asked for more questions per book, so the questions have doubled (200 per book!).
- You wanted questions that better reflect the current format of the Boards, so all questions have been updated to match the current USMLE format for Step 3.
- You liked the detailed explanations for every answer—right or wrong—so we made sure that complete correct and incorrect answers were provided for each question.
- You needed a smaller trim size for easier portability, and now you have it. This edition is small enough to fit in a white coat pocket.
- You were looking for an easier way to test yourself, and we redesigned this edition to do just that. Answer keys and tabbed sections make for easier navigation between questions and answers.
- You wanted an index for easy reference, and you got it (along with abbreviations and normal lab values).

We hope you like this new edition of the Blueprints Q&A series as much as we do. And keep your suggestions and ideas coming! Please send any comments you may have about this book, or any book in the Blueprints series, to *blue@bos.blackwellpublishing.com*.

The Publisher
Blackwell Publishing

Acknowledgments

A heartfelt thanks to Melissa Hardy for her patience, perseverance, and humor assisting with the preparation of the text and to our Psychiatry residents and medical students at Good Samaritan for their inquisitiveness and fresh thinking.

—*James B. McLoone*

Abbreviations

ACE	angiotensin-converting enzyme	HT	serotonin
AD	Alzheimer's disease	ICU	intensive care unit
ADHD	attention deficit hyperactivity disorder	Li	lithium
		LSD	D-lysergic acid
AIDS	acquired immunodeficiency syndrome	MAOI	monoamine oxidase inhibitor
		MDMA	3,4-Methylene dioxymethamphetamine (Ecstasy)
ALT	alanine transaminase		
AMA	American Medical Association		
APOE	apolipoprotein E	MMSE	Mini-Mental Status Exam
AST	aspartate transaminase	MRI	magnetic resonance imaging
AUD	alcohol use disorder	MS	multiple sclerosis
BPD	borderline personality disorder	NE	norepinephrine
BUN	blood urea nitrogen	NMDA	N-methyl-D-aspartate
CBC	complete blood count	NMS	neuroleptic malignant syndrome
CBT	cognitive-behavioral therapy	NSAID	nonsteroidal anti-inflammatory drug
CMP	comprehensive metabolic profile		
CNS	central nervous system	OCD	obsessive-compulsive disorder
CPK	creatine phosphokinase	PCP	phencyclidine, primary care provider
CRF	corticotropin-releasing factor		
CT	computed tomography	PD	Parkinson's disease
DA	dopamine	PET	positron emission tomography
DBT	dialectical behavior therapy	PMDD	premenstrual dysphoric disorder
D_2	dopamine-2	PNS	parasympathetic nervous system
DEA	Drug Enforcement Agency	PPD	purified protein derivative
DID	dissociative identity disorder	PTSD	post-traumatic stress disorder
DLB	dementia with Lewy bodies	REM	rapid eye movement
DSM	*Diagnostic and Statistical Manual of Mental Disorders*	SAD	seasonal affective disorder, social anxiety disorder
DTs	delirium tremens	SDAT	senile dementia, Alzheimer's type
ECT	electroconvulsive therapy	SDRI	selective dopamine reuptake inhibitor
ED	emergency department		
EEG	electroencephalogram	SMI	seriously mentally ill
EKG	electrocardiogram	SNS	sympathetic nervous system
EPS	extrapyramidal symptoms	SPECT	single photon emission computed tomography
FAS	fetal alcohol syndrome		
FDA	Food and Drug Administration	SR	sustained release
FSH	follicle-stimulating hormone	SSRI	selective serotonin reuptake inhibitor
GABA	gamma-aminobutyric acid		
GAD	generalized anxiety disorder	TCA	tricyclic antidepressant
HIPAA	Health Insurance Portability and Accountability Act	TD	tardive dyskinesia
		TSH	thyroid-stimulating hormone
HIV	human immunodeficiency virus		

Questions

Setting 1: Community-Based Health Center

You work at a community-based health facility where patients seeking both routine and urgent care are encountered. Many patients are members of low-income groups; many are ethnic minorities. Several industrial parks and local businesses send their employees to the health center for treatment of on-the-job injuries and employee health screening. There is a facility that provides x-ray films, but CT and MRI scans must be arranged at other facilities. Laboratory services are available.

1. A 54-year-old divorced Hispanic man is being evaluated at the community clinic for daytime sleepiness. His 20-year-old daughter is concerned that her father might have narcolepsy. Symptoms of narcolepsy include which one of the following?

A. Absence-like seizures
B. Cataplexy
C. Catalepsy
D. Snoring
E. Continued tiredness even after napping

2. A 33-year-old divorced mother of three being seen in the community clinic is diagnosed with the rapid-cycling variant of bipolar disorder. Her liver function and renal functions are normal. Which of the following options would be the best initial treatment?

A. Sertraline
B. Paroxetine
C. Lithium
D. Valproic acid
E. Outpatient observation only

3. A 28-year-old waitress is brought to the clinic's urgent care service by her boyfriend after she ingested 10 diazepam tablets. Which of the following medications is the benzodiazepine antagonist used as a possible treatment for benzodiazepine toxicity?

A. Narcan
B. N-acetylcysteine
C. Flumazenil
D. Methadone
E. Temazepam

4. A 32-year-old tile setter with a history of frequent insomnia presents to the clinic's urgent care service with the complaint of a persistent, painful penile erection for the last 5 hours. He is diagnosed with priapism and treated accordingly. Which of the following medications is most likely to have caused this side effect?

A. Bupropion
B. Trazodone
C. Nortriptyline
D. Haloperidol
E. Divalproex sodium

The next two questions (items 5 and 6) correspond to the following vignette.

An 83-year-old retired janitor with a history of hypertension and mild heart failure has been referred by his family physician. Over the past 5 years, the patient has experienced a declining memory and the presumed diagnosis has been senile dementia, Alzheimer's type (SDAT). The patient's PCP initially prescribed donepezil but was required to stop it due to side effects. A trial of rivastigmine was better tolerated and proved helpful until the past 3 months. Increased doses have not made a difference. Presently, the patient's Mini-Mental Status Examination (MMSE) score is 19.

5. In regard to the patient's pharmacologic treatment, which one of the following options is the best step to take next?

    A. Stop the rivastigmine and start galantamine

    B. Add galantamine to the rivastigmine

    C. Add risperidone to the rivastigmine

    D. Add memantine to the rivastigmine

    E. Stop the rivastigmine and start memantine

6. What is the primary mechanism of action of the new medication prescribed to this patient?

    A. Specifically inhibits acetylcholinesterase but not butyrylcholine esterase

    B. Reversibly inhibits actylcholinesterase and butyrylcholine esterase

    C. Acts as an N-methyl-D-aspartate (NMDA) receptor antagonist

    D. Has agonistic effects at the $5HT_3$ receptor

    E. Inhibits acetylcholinesterase and modulates nicotine receptors

End of set

---

7. A 16-year-old high school honors student is being seen in the community clinic's walk-in service for agitation, combativeness, and paranoid thoughts. His speech is rapid, and on exam he has tachycardia with pupillary dilation. His presentation is consistent with which type of substance intoxication?

    A. Heroin

    B. Methamphetamine

    C. Inhalants

    D. Marijuana

    E. Alcohol

8. A 13-year-old gang member with a history of truancy and petty theft is brought to the clinic's urgent care service by police after being arrested for vandalism. He is aggressive and disoriented. Physical exam reveals slurred speech, ataxia, poor motor coordination, and silver stains around his lips. What is the most likely diagnosis?

    A. Bipolar disorder

    B. Conduct disorder

    C. Cocaine intoxication

    D. Acute alcohol ingestion

    E. Inhalant intoxication

9. A 23-year-old law student has been under considerable stress lately while preparing for her final exams. She is brought into the community clinic by her parents because she "can't stop talking." According to her friends, the patient has been extremely hyperactive and productive for the last 5 days. Upon examination, she is smiling, friendly, and talking rapidly. She states that she has been "painting nonstop" without sleep for almost a week because God has chosen her to be the "world's greatest artist!" The triage nurse informs you that the patient's urine drug screen is negative. What is the most likely diagnosis for this patient?

    A. Schizophrenia
    B. Delusional disorder, grandiose type
    C. Bipolar disorder, manic phase
    D. Bipolar disorder, mixed phase
    E. Dissociative identity disorder

The next two questions (items 10 and 11) correspond to the following vignette.

A 33-year-old seriously mentally ill man presents to the clinic's urgent care clinic with urinary retention, tachycardia, mydriasis, and dry skin.

10. Which of the following psychiatric medications is most likely causing this syndrome?

    A. Fluoxetine
    B. Paroxetine
    C. Valproic acid
    D. Alprazolam
    E. Clozapine

11. Which of the following medications is used to reverse the syndrome?

    A. Lorazepam
    B. Physostigmine
    C. Atropine
    D. Thioridazine
    E. Valproic acid

End of set

---

12. An 18-year-old high school senior and body builder is brought to the clinic by his family for "bizarre behavior." Upon examination, the patient is physically agitated and restless, stating that he needs to buy a gun because he believes people are following him. On physical exam, he is noted to be diaphoretic and tachycardic, and has dilated pupils. The patient is guarded and distrustful for most of the interview. His parents state that their son's behavior has become increasingly erratic and distrustful over the last few weeks since he began hanging out with a "bad group of kids." What would be the most appropriate next step in this case?

    A. Admit the patient to the psychiatric unit for observation
    B. Order a CT scan of the brain
    C. Order a urine drug screen

    D. Give the patient 2 mg of intramuscular lorazepam to calm him down
    E. Discharge the patient home if he can contract for safety

13. A 45-year-old special-education teacher with a past history of episodic alcohol abuse complains of being depressed. During an interview, the patient states that for the last 2 years she has felt sad "throughout the day" almost every day, with feelings of low energy, low self-esteem, poor concentration, and decreased appetite. The patient denies any current or past thoughts of harming herself. What is the most likely diagnosis for this patient?

    A. Major depressive disorder, single episode
    B. Major depressive disorder, recurrent
    C. Dysthymic disorder
    D. Cyclothymic disorder
    E. Bipolar disorder, depressed phase

14. A 45-year-old recently separated accountant with two children presents to the clinic with the complaint that he "can't stop worrying." He reports that his work has suffered over the last few weeks because he constantly has to check to make sure he has done everything "just right." The patient admits that his behavior may be excessive, but he is unable to control it. He also complains of several unpleasant, intrusive thoughts of an aggressive nature that he cannot make go away. The patient reports that he stopped driving a car about a week ago because he had to constantly stop and make sure he had not "run anybody over." What is this patient's most likely diagnosis?

    A. Generalized anxiety disorder
    B. Schizophrenia
    C. Delusional disorder
    D. Obsessive-compulsive disorder
    E. Panic disorder

15. A mother brings her 8-year-old son to the clinic because she is concerned about his "bad behavior." For the last year, the child has had problems both at home and at school because of his failure to complete chores and homework. His teachers say that he is unable to sit still or pay attention in class, is easily distracted, and is unable to follow instructions. When asked, his mother responds that her son has never gotten into a fight at school, nor has he been truant or deceitful. The child fidgets in his chair throughout the entire interview. When asked what he thinks is wrong, he replies, "I just get bored real easy." What is this child's most likely diagnosis?

    A. Conduct disorder
    B. Attention deficit hyperactivity disorder
    C. General anxiety disorder
    D. Adjustment disorder with disturbance of conduct
    E. Malingering

16. A 28-year-old single grocery store cashier followed at the community clinic for her bipolar disorder is concerned that she is pregnant and worried about possible birth defects caused by her medication. You tell her that the use of lithium during the first trimester of pregnancy is associated with which teratogenic effect?

  A. Neural tube defect
  B. Ebstein's anomaly
  C. Craniofacial defects
  D. Fingernail hypoplasia
  E. Acromegaly

17. The nurse practitioners at the clinic ask you, the only psychiatrist on staff, to give them an in-service presentation on prescribing psychotropic medications to older patients. Which of the following effects do you tell them is associated with pharmacokinetics and aging?

  A. Volume of distribution increases for lipid-soluble drugs
  B. Volume of distribution increases for water-soluble drugs
  C. Decreased metabolism causes decreased half-lives
  D. Unbound percentage of albumin-bound drugs decreases
  E. Total body weight increases

The following three questions (items 18, 19, and 20) relate to the same clinical scenario.

A 34-year-old public defender presents to his primary care physician's office at the clinic with a complaint of increased stress. He appears to be having difficulty getting to work on time in the morning and reports that he is frequently showing up 2 to 3 hours late despite waking up earlier each day. Increasing time is spent on his morning routine, and he is beginning to recognize it as being excessive. Upon further questioning, the patient remarks that he has been spending most of his morning time trying to avoid contaminating germs. He is neatly dressed but his hands are raw with cracked, dry skin. Otherwise, the physical examination is normal.

18. What is the most likely diagnosis?

  A. Generalized anxiety disorder (GAD)
  B. Paranoid schizophrenia
  C. Delusional disorder
  D. Obsessive-compulsive disorder (OCD)
  E. Hypochondriasis

19. What medication and dosage range would be most effective for this patient over the long term?

  A. Fluoxetine, low dose
  B. Fluoxetine, high dose
  C. Olanzapine, low dose
  D. Olanzapine, high dose
  E. Venlafaxine, low dose

20. The appropriate medication and dosage have been prescribed. When would a clinical response to the medication be expected?

A. Immediately
B. Within 3 days
C. Within 1 to 2 weeks
D. Within 2 to 4 weeks
E. Within 6 to 8 weeks

End of set

The next two questions (items 21 and 22) correspond to the following vignette.

A 40-year-old home health provider is referred by her primary care physician at the clinic for psychiatric consultation. She complains of depression and insists that her husband has been cheating on her. She also thinks that several months ago the front door of her home was painted while she was away. There were paint drops on the floor, and she assumed that her husband's "mistress" had been in the home. The patient has had periods of depression in the past but no hospitalizations. When she is not depressed, she does not have suspicions of her husband's fidelity. She denies auditory or visual hallucinations. The patient works full-time in addition to managing her home. She denies use of illicit drugs or alcohol, and she cannot identify any recent acute stressors. Her MMSE score is 30/30.

21. What is this patient's most likely diagnosis?

A. Major depressive disorder with psychotic features
B. Schizophrenia, paranoid type
C. Adjustment disorder not otherwise specified
D. Schizoaffective disorder
E. Alzheimer's disease

22. The patient has no active medical issues but does admit to a history of binging and purging. What is a possible effective treatment strategy for her current illness?

A. Sertraline and diazepam
B. Fluoxetine
C. Valproic acid
D. SSRI and an antipsychotic
E. Bupropion

23. A 28-year-old art student with a history of sickle cell anemia presents to her community clinic for the first time complaining of "spells" lasting several minutes and leaving her confused. Which of the following symptoms is most typically associated with partial complex seizures?

A. Hemiballism
B. Lacunar states
C. Dissociative phenomena
D. Scanning speech
E. Akathisia

24. A young couple have brought their 6-year-old child to the clinic quite concerned that the youngster has been wetting the bed while asleep at night. Bed-wetting is most typically associated with which of the following characteristics?

    A. Girls
    B. Pathological at age 3
    C. Higher socioeconomic status
    D. Genetic factors
    E. Psychosis

25. After their 8-year-old son refused to go to school 6 days in a row, a perplexed and frustrated couple bring the boy to the community clinic. School phobia is most likely associated with which of the following conditions?

    A. Fire setting
    B. Depression
    C. Enuresis
    D. Learning disabilities
    E. Separation anxiety

End of set

---

26. As the faculty psychiatrist at the community clinic, you have been asked to give the next group of second-year medical students a talk about relaxation therapy. Which one of the following is a specific type of relaxation therapy?

    A. Confrontation
    B. Interpretation
    C. Guided imagery
    D. Self-revelation
    E. Silence

27. Your next talk to the medical students rotating through the clinic will cover the epidemiology of psychiatric illness. Which of the following psychiatric disorders has an equal lifetime prevalence for men and women?

    A. Depression
    B. Seasonal affective disorder (SAD)
    C. Panic disorder
    D. Alcohol dependence
    E. Bipolar disorder

28. The community clinic's advisory board has decided to create a discrete Women's Health Program. The clinic pharmacists have requested that you speak with them about how this development might affect their stocking medications. Which of the following has an essentially equal effect between men and women in terms of the pharmacokinetics of medications?

    A. Hepatic metabolism
    B. Drug absorption
    C. Protein binding
    D. Middle age
    E. Milligram per kilogram (mg per kg) dosing

29. The Women's Health Program has asked that you provide psychiatric consultations to its gynecologic clinic related to premenstrual dysphoric disorder (PMDD). Which of the following is considered the greatest risk factor for PMDD?

A. Clinical depression
B. Postpartum blues
C. OCD
D. Oral contraceptives
E. Panic disorder

30. A 26-year-old woman on parole for shoplifting is seeking pediatric care at the community clinic for her 18-month-old daughter. The mother is concerned about her daughter's development and is worried that her alcohol use during the pregnancy might have damaged the child. Which one of the following is a feature of fetal alcohol syndrome (FAS)?

A. Hypertonia
B. Attention deficit disorder
C. Normal intelligence
D. Growth acceleration
E. Incidence of 1 to 2 cases per 100,000 live births

31. The community clinic has partnered with a nearby halfway house for recovering alcoholics. You are asked to see a 28-year-old woman with a history of hepatitis to establish a primary caregiver relationship with her. Which of the following gender-specific differences related to alcoholism is true?

A. Alcohol dehydrogenase is more active in women
B. Men have relatively higher mortality rates from alcoholism
C. Alcoholism is far less common in young women than in young men
D. Risk factors for alcoholism in women include sexual abuse
E. Alcoholism tends to precede depression in women

32. A 46-year-old divorcee with a history of marijuana use has been prescribed lorazepam through the community clinic routinely for 3 years. Lately she has been asking for more than is called for by her usual dosage schedule. The treatment team members would like to help this patient develop alternative strategies for stress management and wean her off the medication, but are concerned about managing the side effects of withdrawal. Which one of the following statements is true regarding withdrawal from benzodiazepines?

A. Hyperpyrexia, seizures, psychosis, and death can occur in severe withdrawal.
B. Bradycardia, decreased blood pressure, and hypersomnia occur in moderate withdrawal.
C. Withdrawal symptoms typically occur several weeks after discontinuation.
D. Withdrawal typically continues for 3 to 4 days.
E. A reasonable dose reduction rate is 25% per week for patients treated with alprazolam for longer than 2 to 3 months, if discontinuation of the medication is desired.

33. The community mental health clinic has decided to establish a program for patients with panic disorder and agoraphobia that will include educational groups and medication management. Which of the following drugs has been shown to have the best efficacy and tolerance in treating panic disorder?

    A. Selective serotonin reuptake inhibitors (SSRIs)
    B. Tricyclic antidepressants (TCAs)
    C. Beta blockers
    D. Antiarrhythmics
    E. Dilantin

34. Faced with increasing budget constraints, the community mental health center's residential alcohol detoxification program is shifting its resources and clientele to the outpatient clinic. To ensure that medications are stocked appropriately, you need to know that which one of the following is a medication used during the recovery phase to help maintain sobriety?

    A. Disulfiram
    B. Thiamine
    C. Folate
    D. Lorazepam
    E. Chlordiazepoxide

35. During her first postpartum follow-up appointment at the clinic, a 26-year-old woman's husband relates that she has developed symptoms of agitation, labile mood, auditory hallucinations, and paranoia over the 2 weeks following delivery of a healthy baby boy. Which one of the following statements is most accurate regarding postpartum psychosis?

    A. There is no increased incidence with a family history of psychiatric illness.
    B. There is no increased incidence with a history of previous postpartum psychiatric illness.
    C. The incidence is greatest with a history of postpartum blues.
    D. Most episodes occur within the 1 to 2 weeks after delivery.
    E. Overall incidence is 5% to 10% of all deliveries.

36. A 63-year-old widow presents to her primary care physician at the clinic with symptoms of crying, insomnia, and trouble concentrating since the death of her husband 4 weeks earlier. Which one of the following characteristics is most reflective of a normal grieving process?

    A. Survivor guilt
    B. Usually resolves in 2 to 3 months
    C. Is similar throughout all cultures
    D. Decreased vulnerability to physical illness
    E. Is not affected by preparation for the loss

37. The clinic's walk-in substance treatment program continues to be busy. The most popular drugs in the neighborhood lately have been stimulants and alcohol. Which of the following symptoms is associated with amphetamine intoxication?

    A. Depression
    B. Indifference

C. Grandiosity
D. Lethargy
E. Constricted pupils

The next four questions (items 38–41) correspond to the following vignette.

A 33-year-old female presents to her primary care physician's office at the clinic with a chief complaint of a 13-year history of unstable mood and difficulty controlling her anger. Her medical history is unremarkable. Social history is significant for three divorces, a history of alcohol and methamphetamine abuse currently in remission, and difficulty holding the same job for longer than 3 months. Physical exam is significant for multiple lengthwise scars on her wrists. She is dressed in darkly colored, baggy clothing, makes minimal eye contact, and becomes tearful when talking about her symptoms.

38. Which of the following personality disorders does this patient most likely have?

A. Antisocial personality disorder
B. Obsessive-compulsive personality disorder
C. Borderline personality disorder
D. Schizoid personality disorder
E. Histrionic personality disorder

39. Considering the patient's presentation, what would be the most important area of inquiry at this appointment?

A. Depressive symptoms
B. Family history
C. Alcohol use
D. Developmental history
E. Suicidal ideation

40. Over the course of the patient's treatment, which primitive defense mechanism would this patient most likely exhibit?

A. Undoing
B. Splitting
C. Intellectualization
D. Altruism
E. Humor

41. Assuming her diagnosis is correct, what is the preferred method of treatment for this patient's personality disorder?

A. Medication management only
B. Long-term psychotherapy with medication management
C. Short-term therapy only
D. Electroconvulsive therapy (ECT) with medication management
E. There is no appropriate treatment for this condition

End of set

42. A 23-year-old African American graduate student with a history of sarcoidosis presents to the walk-in service of the clinic complaining of "nervousness" for 6 weeks. Upon further examination, she relates a 20-pound weight loss despite a good appetite. On physical examination, her pulse is 130 beats per minute. Which of the following psychiatric symptoms is typically seen in patients with severe hyperthyroidism?

    A. Indifference
    B. Slowed speech
    C. Psychosis
    D. Compulsions
    E. Neologisms

43. The community clinic has a large number of patients with dual diagnoses, often including both schizophrenia and substance abuse. Today, a 43-year-old homemaker is seen in consultation after being referred by her internist, who is concerned about the patient's alcohol consumption and wishes to start her on benzodiazepines to aid in withdrawal. The patient has been diagnosed with paranoid schizophrenia for 15 years. Which of the following statements is true regarding benzodiazepines?

    A. Benzodiazepines provide adequate coverage for heroin withdrawal.
    B. Benzodiazepines function via dopaminergic receptors to cause influx of chloride ions into a cell.
    C. Benzodiazepines are useful in the treatment of catatonia.
    D. Lorazepam and chlordiazepoxide are seldom used for alcohol withdrawal states.
    E. Benzodiazepines may decrease clozapine levels.

44. A 16-year-old high school honors student is reluctantly brought to the clinic by her parents, who are very concerned with their daughter's weight loss, moodiness, and fixation on getting good grades. Which of the following symptoms is typically seen in patients with anorexia nervosa?

    A. Disinterest in food
    B. Binge eating
    C. Premenstrual dysphoria
    D. Diminished appetite
    E. Hypersexuality

45. A 21-year-old liberal arts major was recently hospitalized for her first manic episode. Her hospitalization was complicated by a suicide attempt and a urinary tract infection. She has been referred to the clinic for follow-up care as she tries to finish her last semester of college. She has several poignant questions about potential problems if she continues taking the prescribed lithium. Which of the following is a side effect of lithium?

    A. Weight loss
    B. Leukopenia
    C. Acne
    D. Decreased urine output
    E. Hyperthyroidism

The next three questions (items 46, 47, and 48) correspond to the following vignette.

A 53-year-old woman presents to the clinic's walk-in service with tachycardia, tremor, anxiety, psychomotor agitation, and insomnia.

46. This constellation of symptoms is most closely associated with which of the following conditions?

    A. Alcohol intoxication
    B. Barbiturate intoxication
    C. Barbiturate withdrawal
    D. Benzodiazepine intoxication
    E. Chloral hydrate intoxication

47. What is the standard initial dose for a pentobarbital challenge test?

    A. Pentobarbital 50 mg
    B. Pentobarbital 200 mg
    C. Pentobarbital 400 mg
    D. Pentobarbital 800 mg
    E. Pentobarbital 1000 mg

48. What is the usual daily decrease of the barbiturate dosage to facilitate an uncomplicated withdrawal?

    A. 10% decrease per day
    B. 20% decrease per day
    C. 30% decrease per day
    D. 40% decrease per day
    E. 50% decrease per day

End of set

The next two questions (items 49 and 50) correspond to the following vignette.

A 50-year-old mother of three supported by government disability presents to the clinic with a 15-year history of schizoaffective disorder, bipolar type. She has a history of syncope and has been recently diagnosed with long QT syndrome. She is currently taking the five medications listed in question 49, A–E.

49. Which medication should be stopped?

    A. Divalproex sodium
    B. Clonazepam
    C. Thioridazine
    D. Gabapentin
    E. Diphenhydramine

50. The inappropriate medication has been discontinued. Considering this fact, which medication would be best to start her on?

    A. Lithium carbonate
    B. Risperidone
    C. Benztropine
    D. Nortiptyline
    E. Carbamazepine

End of set

Answer Key

1.	B	18.	D	35.	D
2.	D	19.	B	36.	A
3.	C	20.	E	37.	C
4.	B	21.	C	38.	C
5.	D	22.	D	39.	E
6.	C	23.	E	40.	B
7.	B	24.	A	41.	B
8.	E	25.	D	42.	C
9.	C	26.	C	43.	C
10.	E	27.	E	44.	B
11.	B	28.	E	45.	C
12.	C	29.	A	46.	C
13.	C	30.	B	47.	B
14.	D	31.	D	48.	A
15.	B	32.	A	49.	C
16.	B	33.	A	50.	B
17.	A	34.	A		

1. **B.** Cataplexy is an abrupt paralysis or paresis of skeletal muscles that typically follows awakening, highly emotional experiences (such as anger, surprise, or laughter), and physical exercise. It may be generalized, resulting in collapse, or it may remain isolated to a particular muscle group, resulting in transient loss of function. Duration typically lasts a few minutes, and the patient remains awake during the episode. Afterward, the patient usually regains full function without any impairment. Although cataplexy is the pathognomonic symptom of narcolepsy, it can be elicited in only approximately half of all narcoleptics. Other symptoms of narcolepsy include daytime sleepiness, hypnagogic (just before sleep) or hypnopompic (prior to complete awakening) hallucinations, restless sleep, and sleep paralysis.

A. Seizures are not associated with narcolepsy.

C. Cataplexy should not be confused with catalepsy, the waxy flexibility that may be seen in the catatonic type of schizophrenia.

D. Snoring is often a sign of obstructive sleep apnea, rather than narcolepsy.

E. Narcoleptics typically awaken from naps feeling refreshed.

2. **D.** Valproic acid is a mood-stabilizing medication.

A. Antidepressants such as sertraline would not be used alone in bipolar disorder because they can precipitate a manic episode.

B. Monotherapy with an antidepressant such as paroxetine is not appropriate treatment for bipolar disorder.

C. Although lithium is one of the mainstays of treatment for bipolar disorder, valproic acid appears to be more effective at stabilizing rapid-cycling bipolar disorder. Rapid-cycling mood disorder is diagnosed when an individual with bipolar disorder experiences frequent cycles, defined as four or more mood disturbances per year.

E. It is important to treat these individuals with medication and hospitalization as needed, as the suicide rate in rapid cyclers may be higher than that in non-rapid cyclers.

3. **C.** Flumazenil is a benzodiazepine antagonist approved for the treatment of benzodiazepine overdose and the reversal of benzodiazepine oversedation. This drug binds competitively and reversibly to the GABA-benzodiazepine receptor complex and inhibits the effects of benzodiazepines. Flumazenil may not fully reverse benzodiazepines' inhibitory effects on the hypoxic respiratory drive. Continued monitoring of respiration is necessary. Flumazenil also has a short duration of action and may need to be repeatedly administered to antagonize long-acting benzodiazepines. The drug may induce seizures in patients who are prone to seizures. Caution must also be used due to the risk of causing a seizure from benzodiazepine withdrawal in patients who take benzodiazepines chronically.

A. Narcan is given for opioid toxicity.

B. *N*-acetylcysteine is given for acetaminophen overdose.

D. Methadone is given for long-term maintenance treatment of heroin dependence.

E. Temazepam is a benzodiazepine used primarily as a hypnotic agent.

4. **B.** A number of cases of priapism have been reported in patients taking the antidepressant trazodone.

A. Bupropion, an antidepressant, is not associated with priapism.

C. Nortriptyline, a tricyclic antidepressant, is not associated with priapism.

D. Haloperidol, a typical antipsychotic, is not associated with priapism.

E. Divalproex sodium, or valproic acid, is an anticonvulsant with mood-stabilizing properties. It is not associated with priapism.

5. **D.** Adding memantine to the rivastigmine regimen is the best next step because the two drugs have different mechanisms of action and are usually tolerated together. Memantine is helpful for patients with moderate to severe SDAT, which is indicated by this patient's MMSE score of 19 out of a possible 30.

A, B. Galantamine would not likely be more helpful in combination with rivastigmine or alone for a patient with moderately severe SDAT.

C. Risperidone is an antipsychotic. There is no specific indication for prescribing such a medication to the patient described.

E. Because rivastigmine and memantine have different mechanisms of action, an additive effect should be pursued rather than administration of memantine alone.

6. **C.** Memantine's primary mechanism of action is as a moderate-affinity NMDA receptor antagonist.

A. Donepezil specifically inhibits acetylcholinesterase.

B. Rivastigmine inhibits acetylcholinesterase and butyrylcholine esterase.

D. Memantine has antagonistic effects at the $5HT_3$ receptor.

E. Galantamine inhibits acetylcholinesterase and modulates nicotine receptors.

7. **B.** Methamphetamine is a stimulant. As such, it commonly produces agitation, paranoia, rapid speech, tachycardia, diaphoresis, muscle twitching, and dilated pupils.

A. Heroin intoxication should not cause agitation or combativeness. Intoxication will cause pupillary constriction and sedation. While withdrawal from heroin might have a presentation similar to that seen in this patient, paranoia is not commonly associated with heroin withdrawal or intoxication.

C. Inhalants such as glue or paint thinner may produce aggression, impulsivity, and occasionally psychosis, but usually will not cause pupillary dilation.

D. Marijuana intoxication occasionally will cause paranoia and anxiety, but would not account for pupillary dilation or combativeness.

E. Patients intoxicated with alcohol can display rapid shifts from agitation to mood lability, but they are unlikely to have dilated pupils or paranoid thoughts.

8. **E.** Aromatic hydrocarbons found in products such as gasoline, glue, and paint can be abused through inhalation. In addition to the symptoms observed in this patient, signs of intoxication can include grandiosity, euphoria, and visual disturbances. The silver stains are likely from inhaling spray paint.

A. Bipolar disorder would not account for the physical exam findings in this patient.

B. Conduct disorder would not account for the physical findings in this patient.

C. Cocaine intoxication might cause impulsivity and aggression, but would not cause slurred speech or ataxia.

D. Alcohol can cause mood lability, irritability, slurred speech, ataxia, and motor incoordination, but would not account for the silver stains around this patient's mouth.

9. **C.** This patient is exhibiting symptoms of an acute manic episode of a bipolar disorder: acute hyperactivity, pressured speech, psychomotor agitation with goal-oriented activity, decreased need for sleep, and mood elevation to the point of developing a delusion of grandeur. Her negative drug screen helps eliminate the possibility of substance-induced mania or psychotic behavior.

A. The patient does not exhibit enough symptoms consistent with a diagnosis of schizophrenia (e.g., auditory or visual hallucinations, ideas of reference, thought blocking, thought insertion, avolition, catatonia).

B. Although the patient does indeed have a grandiose delusion, the diagnosis of delusional disorder would not explain her other symptoms such as pressured speech and increased psychomotor activity.

D. The patient is neither complaining nor exhibiting any symptoms of depression; therefore, this is likely not a mixed phase of mania.

E. No evidence indicates that this patient's symptoms are due to dissociative states or multiple personalities.

10. **E.** Clozapine is an antipsychotic medication with potent anticholinergic effects. It is typically reserved for use in seriously mentally ill patients with chronic persistent symptoms.

A. Fluoxetine has essentially no anticholinergic properties.

B. Paroxetine has minimal anticholinergic properties.

C. Valproic acid has no anticholinergic properties.

D. Alprazolam has no anticholinergic properties.

11. **B.** Physostigmine reverses the syndrome by inhibiting acetylcholinesterase, the enzyme that breaks down acetylcholine.

A. Lorazepam and other benzodiazepines may calm the agitated patient but will not reverse the condition.

C. Atropine, as an anticholinergic agent, would worsen the condition.

D. Thioridazine and other typical antipsychotics have anticholinergic effects.

E. Valproic acid is an anticonvulsant with mood-stabilizing properties but would not be helpful in this patient.

12. C. It would be extremely helpful at this time to determine what is causing the patient's symptoms, whether a primary psychiatric condition (schizophrenia) or an organic condition (substance-induced psychosis). The patient's physical exam findings and his parents' information suggest that this is likely a stimulant-induced psychotic episode.

A. Admitting the patient is not the best option at this time. He currently needs a more thorough medical evaluation (i.e., urine drug screen, possible head CT). If this is indeed a substance-induced psychosis, his symptoms may diminish after a period of detoxification.

B. Ordering a CT scan is not the most appropriate step at this time. It would be more prudent to await the results of the urine drug screen before ordering additional tests. If the drug screen is negative, then a CT of the brain may be warranted, especially if the patient has a history of recent head trauma.

D. The patient is restless and agitated but is not currently threatening or combative. Lorazepam can be given at any time if needed.

E. It would be inappropriate to discharge this patient until a diagnosis has been made and a thorough risk assessment of his suicidal and homicidal status has been performed. Currently, this patient is paranoid and is talking about buying a gun. His symptoms may improve over a short time course if this is a substance-induced disorder, but discharge at this time is premature. It is likely that he will require admission.

13. C. The chronology and intensity of the patient's symptoms are consistent with the diagnostic criteria for dysthymic disorder (feeling depressed most of the day, more days than not, for a period of at least 2 years).

A, B. Although the symptoms of depressed mood, low energy, low self-esteem, poor appetite, and decreased sleep are found in both major depressive disorder and dysthymic disorder, the consistency and length of this patient's symptoms are more diagnostic of dysthymic disorder than a major depressive disorder, single or recurrent. No evidence suggests a recurrent or episodic condition.

D. The patient has not exhibited any current or past symptoms of hypomania, which would be required for a diagnosis of cyclothymic disorder.

E. A history of mania would be required to make a diagnosis of bipolar disorder.

14. D. Obsessive-compulsive disorder is the correct answer. The patient has both obsessions and compulsions that he recognizes are excessive and are causing him marked distress.

A. The patient is not complaining of constant anxiety over numerous life events, which would be necessary to make a diagnosis of GAD.

B. This patient does not have hallucinations, delusions, disorganized speech, catatonic behavior, or any of the other major symptoms typical of schizophrenia.

C. This patient is not really delusional, seemingly appreciating an irrationality to his excessive worrying and unusual behavior.

E. This patient does not describe a history of panic attacks, which would be required to make a diagnosis of panic disorder.

15. **B.** This child has attention deficit hyperactivity disorder (ADHD). He has had problems for more than 6 months at two different settings in regard to paying attention, sitting still, being easily distracted, following instructions, and demonstrating hyperactivity. These symptoms are severe enough to have caused him impaired functioning both at home and in school.

A. The patient does not have a history of truancy from school, fighting, or deceitfulness, so a diagnosis of conduct disorder is inappropriate.

C. The patient complains of boredom and his symptoms are marked by distractibility and hyperactivity, not anxiety.

D. No identifiable stressor has occurred within the last 3 months that would account for the child's behavior. Also, the patient's symptoms have been present for longer than 1 year.

E. There are no external incentives or secondary gains to explain this child's behavior.

16. **B.** Ebstein's anomaly is a serious cardiac defect involving the tricuspid valve. First-trimester use of lithium increases the risk to 1/1000 from 1/20,000 in the general population.

A. Neural tube defects are associated with valproic acid and carbamazepine exposure during pregnancy.

C. Craniofacial defects are associated with valproic acid and carbamazepine exposure during pregnancy.

D. Fingernail hypoplasia is associated with valproic acid and carbamazepine exposure during pregnancy.

E. Acromegaly is a condition associated with pituitary tumors and excessive levels of growth hormone.

17. **A.** There is an increase in total body fat with aging, especially in women.

B. The volume of distribution for water-soluble drugs decreases with aging.

C. The decreases in renal blood flow and hepatic enzyme activity associated with aging result in decreased metabolism rates and, therefore, longer half-lives for medications.

D. Albumin decreases with aging, so the unbound percentage increases.

E. Typically the elderly experience a decrease in total body weight, which affects milligram per kilogram prescribing.

18. | **D.** OCD is characterized by obsessions, compulsions, or both. This patient engages in compulsive hand washing and cleaning rituals to avoid contamination. The diagnosis of OCD also requires that he recognize the symptoms as being excessive and that they produce noticeable interference with his usual functioning.

A. GAD might be a consideration, but the presence of specific obsessions and compulsions is better explained by OCD.

B. This patient does not exhibit any symptoms of psychosis, which makes a diagnosis of schizophrenia unlikely.

C. Delusional disorder is unlikely because the patient is not psychotic.

E. Patients with hypochondriasis usually do not try to resist their thoughts of contamination, nor do they think them unreasonable.

19. | **B.** The most effective medications for OCD are SSRIs such as fluoxetine, and higher doses are typically required.

A. The lower dose of fluoxetine might be started, but the dosage goal would be approximately 60 to 80 mg per day.

C, D. There is no evidence supporting the use of the atypical antipsychotic olanzapine at any dose for OCD.

E. A mixed serotonin/norepinephrine reuptake inhibitor such as venlafaxine might be efficacious for OCD (although it is not approved for this use), but the goal would likely be a higher dose to achieve a sufficient serotonin effect.

20. | **E.** The bulk of scientific evidence on treating OCD with SSRIs supports the notion that a delayed response is the rule. A response would be expected in 6 to 8 weeks at the earliest, but it might take several months to achieve clinical improvement. When used to treat depression, SSRIs typically produce improvements in 3 to 5 weeks. An earlier response might be seen in either illness, but it is no more likely than with placebo.

A, B, C, D. An expected time frame for a medication response for OCD is not less than 6 to 8 weeks.

21. | **A.** The patient most likely has a major depressive disorder with psychosis.

B. The significant mood component and the fact that she does not exhibit a typical picture of schizophrenia (e.g., early age of onset and chronic deteriorating clinical course) make schizophrenia an unlikely diagnosis in this patient.

C. There is no identifiable acute stressor that would lead to an adjustment disorder.

D. To make a diagnosis of schizoaffective disorder, there would have to be a significant period during which psychotic symptoms existed in the absence of mood symptoms.

E. The patient's age makes dementia unlikely. Furthermore, she shows no evidence of cognitive decline.

22. **D.** The patient requires an antidepressant, most likely an SSRI, for her mood disorder as well as an antipsychotic for her delusional perceptions.

A. Sertraline and the anxiolytic diazepam would not likely sufficiently treat her psychosis.

B. Fluoxetine alone would not likely treat her psychosis adequately.

C. Valproic acid is a mood stabilizer that is effective in treating bipolar disorder and may also be effective in treating schizoaffective disorder. It would not be effective in treating this patient's depression or depression-related psychosis.

E. The patient should not be prescribed bupropion due to her history of an eating disorder and the increased risk of seizures in such individuals who take bupropion.

23. **C.** Partial complex seizures may cause prolonged dissociative states resembling catatonia.

A. Hemiballism involves unilateral involuntary movement typical of chorea.

B. Lacunar states are the pathological findings in the brain associated with atherosclerosis.

D. Scanning speech is a nonspecific abnormality associated with conditions such as multiple sclerosis.

E. Akathisia is a subjective experience of jitteriness and difficulty remaining still that is typically seen as a side effect of antipsychotic medications.

24. **D.** Bed-wetting runs in families, typically in fathers and sons.

A. Bed-wetting, or enuresis, is much more common in boys.

B. Bed-wetting is pathological if it occurs repeatedly in someone at least 5 years old and is not caused by a physical condition or medication.

C. For reasons that remain unclear, but perhaps are related to stress, bed-wetting is more common in institutionalized children and children of lower socioeconomic status.

E. Psychosis itself is not associated with bed-wetting. Psychological stresses such as birth of a sibling, moving, and parents divorcing may exacerbate bed-wetting.

25. **E.** Children with separation anxiety fear that something bad will happen to them or their caretakers while they are at school.

A. Fire setting, or pyromania, can be seen in school-aged children but is not associated with school phobia.

B. Depression reduces energy and motivation and may dampen a desire to attend school, but it is not the condition most commonly associated with school phobia.

C. Enuresis may cause embarrassment in school so that children want to stay away, but it is not the condition most commonly associated with school phobia.

D. Learning disabilities often bring ridicule from other students and prompt children to want to stay away from school, but they are less common than separation anxiety as an associated condition.

26. **C.** Guided imagery is a specific relaxation-inducing technique. The patient is coached to visually imagine a relaxing, serene setting as a strategy to reduce stress and anxiety.

A. Confrontation is an aspect of psychotherapy that helps in the interview process by breaking through the defense of denial.

B. Interpretation is an aspect of psychotherapy that helps clarify conflicts.

D. Self-revelation is an aspect of psychotherapy that may help unmask a patient's hidden concerns.

E. Silence fosters contemplation but also tends to create anxiety for the patient.

27. **E.** Bipolar disorder is essentially equally prevalent in men (0.7) and women (0.9). This holds true for bipolar types I and II.

A. The lifetime prevalence of depression in men and women is 12% versus 20%, respectively.

B. The lifetime prevalence of SAD in men and women is 1% versus 6%, respectively.

C. The lifetime prevalence of panic disorder in men and women is 2% versus 5%, respectively.

D. The lifetime prevalence of alcohol dependence in men and women is 20% versus 6%, respectively.

28. **E.** Despite the various possible pharmacokinetic gender-related differences between men and women, a standardized mg per kg dosing approach serves either sex well.

A. Estrogen has an inhibitory effect on some hepatic enzymes.

B. Progesterone can delay gastric emptying and subsequently absorption.

C. Both estrogen and progesterone are protein bound and may compete with medications for binding sites.

D. Case reports suggest that hormonal fluctuations associated with menopause affect medication levels as well.

29. **A.** Clinical depression is highly correlated with PMDD. Although no single cause of PMDD has been established, fluctuations of normal levels of reproductive hormones appear to promote psychological symptoms in susceptible women. Specific symptoms seen in PMDD include depression, anxiety, emotional lability, trouble concentrating, and lethargy.

B. Postpartum blues are not associated with PMDD.

C. OCD has no direct causative relationship to PMDD.

D. Oral contraceptives, especially when continued through the menstrual cycle, may alleviate PMDD.

E. Panic disorder itself does not cause PMDD, but panic episodes may be more frequent premenstrually.

30. | **B.** Attention deficit disorder, with or without hyperactivity, is often manifested in childhood as a feature of FAS.

A. Hypotonia is often present at birth in babies with FAS.

C. Cognitive deficits, including intellectual deficiencies and other learning disabilities, are associated with FAS.

D. FAS is associated with growth retardation.

E. FAS is a relatively common occurrence; even occasional consumption of alcohol may result in fetal defects. The incidence is 1 to 2 cases per 1000 live births.

31. | **D.** Sexual abuse is a risk factor for alcoholism.

A. Alcohol dehydrogenase, the enzyme that breaks down alcohol, is less active in women and likely causes women to more readily become intoxicated.

B. Alcohol-related medical complications occur more quickly in women.

C. Although the overall prevalence of alcoholism among women is much less than among men, this discrepancy is becoming less pronounced in the younger age groups.

E. Mood disorders frequently precede alcoholism in women.

32. | **A.** Hyperpyrexia, seizures, psychosis, and even death can be seen in benzodiazepine withdrawal.

B. Tachycardia, increased blood pressure, and insomnia occur in moderate withdrawal from benzodiazepines.

C. Withdrawal symptoms can occur as soon as the day after discontinuation of benzodiazepines.

D. Withdrawal symptoms can continue for weeks to months after stopping a benzodiazepine.

E. For patients treated with benzodiazepines for longer than 2 to 3 months, a typical dose reduction rate would be 5% to 10% per week. The faster the benzodiazepine's onset of action, the slower the taper should be.

33. | **A.** SSRIs are the most efficacious and well-tolerated agents for the long-term treatment of panic disorder.

B. TCAs are useful in the long-term treatment of panic disorder but are not as well tolerated as SSRIs.

C. Beta blockers have shown limited efficacy in the acute treatment of panic disorder but are not as efficacious as SSRIs for long-term treatment.

D. Antiarrhythmics are not used to treat panic disorder.

E. Although some anticonvulsants have shown efficacy in the treatment of panic disorder, dilantin is not one of them.

34. **A. Disulfiram promotes sobriety by accumulating acetaldehyde and producing very unpleasant physical effects when combined with alcohol.**

B. Thiamine deficiency can occur in chronic alcohol abuse, resulting in Wernicke's encephalopathy. Thiamine is prescribed during the withdrawal phase of treatment.

C. Folate deficiency is common in chronic alcohol abuse, resulting in neurologic symptoms if left untreated. Folate does not help with sobriety.

D. Lorazepam is a short-acting benzodiazepine used to minimize withdrawal symptoms and seizures.

E. Chlordiazepoxide is a longer-acting benzodiazepine used to minimize withdrawal symptoms and seizures.

35. **D. Most postpartum psychotic episodes occur relatively soon after delivery.**

A. Inquiring about a family history of psychiatric illness with special consideration being paid to incidence of bipolar disorder and postpartum psychosis may identify a higher risk.

B. A patient with a previous history of postpartum psychiatric illness should be educated and monitored for a recurrence.

C. All affective disorders, but bipolar disorder in particular, may be manifested for the first time postpartum.

E. Postpartum psychosis is a relatively rare disorder and occurs after 0.1% to 0.2% of all pregnancies.

36. **A. Blaming oneself for how the deceased was treated is common in normal grieving.**

B. Normal grieving is self-limited, but commonly persists for 6 to 12 months.

C. Grieving is manifested differently from culture to culture, so the clinician must be mindful of what is appropriate for the patient.

D. The increased vulnerability to physical illness should be monitored and may allow for follow-up visits for supportive therapy.

E. The course of grieving is affected by the abruptness of the loss.

37. **C. Grandiosity is a behavioral effect associated with amphetamine intoxication.**

A. Depression, fatigue, and hypersomnia are characteristic of amphetamine withdrawal, rather than intoxication.

B. Hypervigilance, rather than indifference, is a behavioral effect associated with amphetamine intoxication.

D. Agitation, rather than lethargy, is a behavioral effect associated with amphetamine intoxication.

E. Dilated pupils, tachycardia, and hypertension are physical effects caused by amphetamines.

38. | **C.** The diagnostic traits of borderline personality disorder seen in this patient include a pattern of unstable relationships, impulsivity (substance abuse), chronic self-destructive behavior, affective instability, and intense anger.

A. The patient does not show the pattern of disregard for the law and lack of remorse seen in antisocial personality disorder.

B. There is no evidence of perfectionism, preoccupation with rules, or moral inflexibility as would be seen in obsessive-compulsive personality disorder.

D. Schizoid personality disorder is unlikely because the patient does not report engagement in solitary activities, emotional detachment, or flattened affect. On the contrary, she reports excessive mood reactivity, and her desire to have close relationships is evidenced by her multiple divorces.

E. If this patient had histrionic personality disorder, she would likely be using her appearance to draw attention to herself or to appear seductive.

39. | **E.** Suicidal ideation. Long-term data on borderline personality disorder indicate a lifetime suicide rate exceeding 5%. The scars on this patient's wrists indicate prior self-mutilation or suicide attempts.

A, B, C, D. While it would be helpful to inquire about depressive symptoms, family history, current alcohol use, and developmental history, the single most important thing to assess in this patient would be dangerousness to herself or to others.

40. | **B.** Examples of primitive defenses include splitting, denial, projection, dissociation, and acting out. The personality disorders—particularly borderline personality disorder—are characterized by use of these more primitive defense mechanisms. Splitting can be described as black-and-white thinking, such as treating someone as if that person were all evil or all good. This consideration is relevant here because this patient may eventually come to view her physician, nurse, or other office staff as all good or all evil.

A. Undoing is considered a "neurotic defense" and might be seen in patients with an anxiety disorder.

C. Intellectualization is another "neurotic defense."

D. Altruism is a mature defense mechanism commonly observed in a psychologically healthy person.

E. Humor is a mature defense mechanism.

41. | **B.** The standard of care for a patient with borderline personality disorder is long-term psychotherapy with adjunctive use of medications for treatment of co-morbid Axis I disorders.

A. Medication management alone may be helpful to some degree, but more significant gains would be expected with concomitant psychotherapy.

C. Personality disorders may initially respond to short-term therapy, but long-standing dysfunctional patterns are likely to return after therapy ends.

D. While ECT may treat an underlying severe mood or persistent psychotic disorder, it is generally not indicated for the treatment of personality disorders.

E. Although often challenging, psychotherapy and prudent use of medications as the borderline patient matures can produce rewarding results.

42. | **C.** More severe hyperthyroidism can result in psychotic symptoms of hallucinations and delusions.

A. Irritability, rather than passivity or indifference, is one of the many mood and personality changes experienced with hyperthyroidism.

B. Hyperthyroidism may be manifested as an energy disorder with rapid speech, racing thoughts, and increased activity.

D. Compulsions are not psychiatric symptoms typically associated with hyperthyroidism, although generalized anxiety is commonly experienced.

E. Neologisms involve the creation of novel words, a behavior sometimes manifested by patients with schizophrenia.

43. | **C.** Benzodiazepines are often used to treat catatonia.

A. Benzodiazepines do not provide adequate coverage for opioid withdrawal. Agents like methadone are more appropriate.

B. Benzodiazepine receptors are closely linked with the GABA receptor. Activity at the benzodiazepine receptor potentiates the action of GABA. This major inhibitory neurotransmitter causes chloride channels to open, allowing influx of chloride into the cell to occur.

D. For a patient in alcohol withdrawal, lorazepam is sometimes preferred to chlordiazepoxide if the patient has liver disease or is elderly, due to the former agent's brief half-life. Both drugs are efficacious, however.

E. Benzodiazepines must be used with caution in patients on clozapine, as they may cause clozapine levels to rise.

44. | **B.** Individuals with anorexia typically eat secretively and often binge.

A. Patients with anorexia nervosa have a preoccupation with food.

C. Starvation commonly produces menstrual irregularities leading to amenorrhea.

D. Despite the use of the term "anorexia," diminished appetite is not the rule in these patients.

E. Loss of sexual interest, decreased alertness, and social withdrawal may occur in conjunction with the starvation of anorexia nervosa.

45. | **C.** Dermatologic side effects from lithium include acne and hair loss.

A. Presumably related to carbohydrate craving and lowered metabolism, lithium frequently causes weight gain.

B. Lithium commonly produces leukocytosis rather than leukopenia.

D. Increased thirst and decreased ability to concentrate follow from lithium-related polyuria.

E. Hypothyroidism is a potential side effect of lithium and is more often seen in women taking lithium than in men.

46. | **C.** Barbiturate and similarly acting sedative, hypnotic, anxiolytic, and alcohol withdrawal syndromes present with similar symptoms. Nausea, vomiting, hallucinations, illusions, and seizures may also develop.

A, B, D, E. Intoxication with alcohol, barbiturates, benzodiazepines, and sedative-hypnotics such as chloral hydrate would result in slurred speech, incoordination, nystagmus, and stupor.

47. | **B.** Pentobarbital 200 mg is given orally, and the patient is observed for intoxication after 1 hour. If not intoxicated, the patient is given another 100 mg every 2 hours, up to a maximum of 500 mg over 6 hours.

A, C, D, E. These are incorrect dosages. See the explanation for B.

48. | **A.** A decrease of approximately 10% per day typically allows for an uncomplicated withdrawal, but the rate must be adjusted if the patient shows signs of intoxication or withdrawal.

B, C, D, E. Decreasing barbiturate doses more than 10% per day could result in a medically dangerous withdrawal state characterized by seizures, psychosis, and even death.

49. | **C.** Thioridazine is an antipsychotic that has been found to cause significant increases in the corrected QT interval. It is absolutely contraindicated in patients with long QT syndrome.

A. Divalproex sodium is not known to cause increases in the QTc.

B. Clonazepam is not known to cause increases in the QTc.

D. Gabapentin is not known to cause increases in the QTc.

E. Diphenhydramine is not known to cause increases in the QTc.

50. | **B.** As an antipsychotic medication, risperidone would be an appropriate replacement for thioridazine. It is not known to cause significant alterations in EKG parameters.

A. Lithium carbonate should not be used in a patient with arrhythmias, and it would not be an effective replacement for an antipsychotic.

C. Benztropine is an anticholinergic medication commonly used to treat extrapyramidal side effects of antipsychotics. It would not be an effective replacement for an antipsychotic.

D. Nortriptyline is a tricyclic antidepressant that may cause tachycardia; it would be contraindicated in a patient with bipolar disorder.

E. Carbamazepine is an anticonvulsant that may be used adjunctively as a mood stabilizer. It would not be an effective replacement for an antipsychotic.

Questions

Setting 2: Office

Your office is in a primary care generalist group practice located in a physician office suite adjoining a suburban community hospital. Patients are usually seen by appointment. Most of the patients you see are from your own practice and are appearing for regular scheduled return visits, with some new patients as well. As in most group practices, you will often encounter a patient whose primary care is managed by one of your associates; reference may be made to the patient's medical records. You may do some telephone management, and you may have to respond to questions about articles in magazines and on television that will require interpretation. Complete laboratory and radiology services are available.

The next three questions (items 51, 52, and 53) correspond to the following vignette.

An 83-year-old widow is accompanied to your office by her daughter, with whom she lives. On examination, the patient is pleasant and attentive, and she denies any specific psychiatric symptoms except for some trouble with her memory. Her Mini-Mental State Examination (MMSE) score is 23.

51. Which of the following medications would be the most appropriate choice for this patient?

    A. Lorazepam
    B. Risperidone
    C. Buspirone
    D. Donepezil
    E. Sertraline

52. Over the course of 2 months, the patient's MMSE score improves to 26, then it plateaus. You increase the medication dose, but she soon complains that the side effects are intolerable. What should be your next step?

    A. Reduce the medication to the earlier dose
    B. Switch to rivastigmine
    C. Add risperidone
    D. Add sertraline
    E. Inform the patient and her daughter that nothing more can be done

53. Over the course of time, your patient's Alzheimer's disease (AD) progresses such that she becomes increasingly paranoid and is experiencing auditory hallucinations. Which of the following statements about antipsychotic medication usage by elderly patients such as this woman is true?

    A. Elderly patients are at increased risk for developing extrapyramidal symptoms (EPS).
    B. Olanzepine does not cause diabetes in the elderly.
    C. Quetiapine does not cause triglyceride elevations in the elderly.
    D. Weight gain is not seen when using atypical antipsychotics in the elderly.
    E. Elderly patients are at less risk for developing anticholinergic side effects.

End of set

---

54. A patient referred to your outpatient office has been self-medicating with herbs and vitamins and asks for your advice on any possible drug interactions. Of the following, which complementary or alternative medicine is most appropriate for a patient with rapid-cycling bipolar disorder?

    A. Kava
    B. Fish oils containing omega 3 fatty acids
    C. Valerian
    D. St. John's wort
    E. Gingko biloba

55. A 68-year-old retired teacher with hypertension is followed in your office. He is otherwise in good health but expresses concern about his sexual performance. You counsel him that which of the following statements is most correct regarding sexuality and normal aging?

   A. Libido generally decreases with age for men and women.
   B. In men, decreased levels of testosterone and follicle-stimulating hormone (FSH) affect libido.
   C. In women, decreased estrogen levels and increased testosterone levels reduce libido.
   D. Few people older than 65 years have a chronic disease that may affect sexual function.
   E. Most men in their seventies report erectile dysfunction.

> The next two questions (items 56 and 57) correspond to the following vignette.

A 16-year-old high school student is referred to your outpatient practice. When you ask her to describe her problems, she relates that she breaks into a cold sweat at supermarket checkout counters and most any other casual social activity. You diagnose her with social anxiety disorder (SAD).

56. Which of the following statements regarding SAD is true?

   A. SAD often begins early in life.
   B. Males are affected more often than females.
   C. SAD is an uncommon disorder.
   D. The majority of individuals with SAD suffer from the nongeneralized type.
   E. Recovery without treatment is common.

57. Which of the following pharmacologic treatments may be helpful for this patient's SAD?

   A. Sertraline
   B. Amitriptyline
   C. Imipramine
   D. Nortriptyline
   E. Desipramine

End of set

58. A 73-year-old retired printer with a history of depression, a movement disorder, and progressive dementia is being followed in your outpatient office practice. Which of the following statements is most true about dementia?

   A. Dementia with Lewy bodies (DLB) accounts for one-fifth of all dementias.
   B. Few patients with DLB experience extrapyramidal symptoms.
   C. Neuroimaging is not helpful to differentiate the various forms of dementia.
   D. Few patients with Parkinson's disease (PD) experience cognitive impairment.
   E. The prevalence of Alzheimer's disease decreases after age 80.

59. A well-groomed, attractive, 38-year-old Hispanic female comes to your outpatient office. She is complaining of stress related to the break-up of her 15-year relationship with the father of her two children. Three months ago her boyfriend went to Mexico, and when he returned he announced that he had married a woman whom he had met just 9 days earlier. Since receiving this news, the patient has experienced initial insomnia, poor energy, and depressed mood for most of the day nearly every day. She has been unable to concentrate in the classes she is taking to become a beautician. However, she continues to enjoy spending time with her two children. The patient denies feelings of guilt, any thoughts of death, or wanting to hurt herself or others. She is anxious about how she will support herself and her children. She has no previous psychiatric history. The patient visits her primary care physician for annual check-ups and has no history of physical illness. She remains composed until the end of the interview, when she becomes tearful and asks, "Doctor, do you think he ever loved me?" Which of the following is her most likely diagnosis?

A. Major depressive disorder, first episode
B. Dysthymia
C. Adjustment disorder, chronic type, with depressed mood
D. Adjustment disorder, acute type, with mixed anxiety and depressed mood
E. Post-traumatic stress disorder

The next two questions (items 60 and 61) correspond to the following vignette.

A 33-year-old woman presents to your office with signs and symptoms of a major depressive episode, recurrent, and without psychotic features. You plan to prescribe an antidepressant medication.

60. Which of the labeled dose-response curves in Figure 60 demonstrates a "therapeutic window" effect for antidepressant medication?

A. Curve A
B. Curve B
C. Curve C
D. Curve D

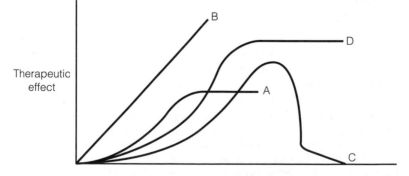

Figure 60

61. A "therapeutic window" dose-response curve is most typically associated with which of the following antidepressants?

A. Desipramine
B. Nortriptyline
C. Fluoxetine
D. Paroxetine
E. Risperidone

End of set

62. A 30-year-old receptionist with a history of premenstrual dysphoric disorder (PMDD) and lupus survives a serious car accident without any physical injuries. In the week immediately following the accident, she is seen for follow-up care at your office. She has developed feelings of detachment, does not remember details about the accident, and appears to be in a daze. She tells you that she is having nightmares about cars and has been unable to go to work for 1 week. What is her most likely diagnosis?

A. Post-traumatic stress disorder (PTSD)
B. Depersonalization disorder
C. Malingering
D. Generalized anxiety disorder
E. Acute stress disorder

63. A 36-year-old flight attendant is referred to your outpatient office practice for assessment and treatment of her refractory depression. Her PCP has prescribed a variety of SSRIs with only moderate success. Which of the following antidepressant combinations or potentiators is most appropriate?

A. Fluoxetine plus sertraline
B. Sertraline plus bupropion
C. Sertraline plus nardil
D. Imipramine plus nardil
E. Lithium plus nardil

The next two questions (items 64 and 65) correspond to the following vignette.

A PCP has asked you to assess his 36-year-old male patient for depression in your outpatient office. The patient's symptoms include fatigue, depressed mood, irritability, sleep disturbance, and poor concentration. To rule out possible medical causes of his symptoms, you pay close attention to the symptoms review portion of the history.

64. Which of the following statements is most likely correct?

A. Inquiring about endocrinologic review of systems is irrelevant.
B. Inquiring about hematologic review of systems is irrelevant.
C. Inquiring about neurologic review of systems is irrelevant.
D. Inquiring about dermatologic review of systems is irrelevant.
E. Inquiring about infectious disease review of systems is irrelevant.

65. Thorough history and exam are performed on the patient to rule out physical causes for his symptoms, and you correctly diagnose him with major depressive disorder. You decide to initiate treatment with paroxetine, as he had taken another SSRI in the past. You carefully educate the patient about which side effect that is especially associated with this medication?

A. Dry mouth
B. Rapid discontinuation syndrome
C. Nausea
D. Headache
E. Delayed ejaculation

End of set

> **The next two questions (items 66 and 67) correspond to the following vignette.**

A 35-year-old hotel concierge presents to your outpatient office. He has a longstanding history of HIV infection and is concerned about new psychiatric symptoms.

66. Which of the following statements regarding the psychiatric manifestations of HIV infection is true?

A. Short-term memory is almost always more affected than long-term memory.
B. Hallucinations are symptoms of a separate primary psychiatric disorder.
C. Opportunistic infections will not cause new psychiatric symptoms.
D. Antiretroviral drug side effects are not a likely cause of new psychiatric symptoms.
E. Neuropsychological testing is unnecessary.

67. During your evaluation of the patient, he admits to hearing voices recently. You suspect auditory hallucinations and recognize the importance of following up on this symptom. Which is the most appropriate follow-up question?

A. Is the voice male or female?
B. Are the voices telling you to do anything?
C. How does that make you feel?
D. Would you allow me to refer you to a psychiatrist?
E. Are you remembering to take your medications?

End of set

---

68. A 49-year-old man followed in your outpatient practice relates that he "hates himself" because he has been secretly dressing in women's underwear for years. The patient adds that he has successfully concealed this practice from everyone, including his wife and children. He finds this behavior "disgusting" and has tried to stop it, but cannot resist the sexual arousal associated with it. Which of the following interventions is the most appropriate for this patient?

A. Discuss the possibility of sexual reassignment surgery
B. Initiate treatment with medroxyprogesterone
C. Have the patient explore the reasons why he finds the behavior disgusting

D. Tell the patient that many men participate in this behavior

E. Suggest that the patient disclose his behavior to his wife and begin marital counseling

69. A 12-year-old boy with a history of truancy is referred by his pediatrician for consideration of antidepressant treatment. The boy is accompanied to your office by his mother and stepfather. Which of the following statements is true regarding mood disorders in children and adolescents?

A. The prevalence of depression in children approaches 1 in 10.

B. The prevalence of depression in adolescents decreases as they approach adulthood.

C. The male to female ratio for depression is 1:1 in childhood.

D. Tricyclics are the antidepressants of choice for younger patients.

E. Antidepressant dosage should be halved upon achieving symptom control in younger patients.

The next three questions (items 70, 71, and 72) correspond to the following vignette.

A 68-year-old retired physician has been referred for outpatient consultation by his neurologist. The patient experienced a stroke 3 months ago but except for daytime somnolence and fatigue has no significant sequelae. The patient's neurologist wonders whether he is depressed, but you discern no specific symptoms to warrant that diagnosis.

70. Which of the following medications is best indicated?

A. Sertraline

B. Ziprasidone

C. Modafinil

D. Carbamazepine

E. Rivastigmine

71. The patient's spouse, who is a retired nurse, asks you how the medication you prescribed works. What is the best description of its mechanism of action?

A. It is a selective serotonin reuptake inhibitor (SSRI)

B. It is a dopamine-receptor blocking agent

C. It prevents reuptake of dopamine

D. It enhances release of GABA

E. It stabilizes neuronal membranes

72. The patient's spouse also questions you about side effects associated with the medication. Which of the following statements is correct?

A. Symptoms of withdrawal are common after several weeks of use.

B. Extra caution is not necessary while driving.

C. It can precipitate symptoms of depression.

D. It does not affect levels of other medications metabolized by the liver.

E. The patient's blood pressure should be monitored.

End of set

The next two questions (items 73 and 74) correspond to the following vignette.

A 48-year-old house painter is referred to you by his family practitioner for complaints of anxiety related to "kidney problems." Despite a thorough evaluation and his PCP's reassurance that there is no evidence of disease, the patient is convinced he is "going to die in the next 10 years" from kidney disease. A typical episode of anxiety begins when he starts to feel warm when he is working, followed by shortness of breath. He starts to worry about his blood pressure rising and his kidneys malfunctioning, leading to a build-up of toxins. His PCP prescribed citalopram initially, but the patient believed that it made his "breathing" worse so he discontinued it. His PCP then prescribed clonazepam, which helps his anxiety. The patient admits that he sometimes takes an extra afternoon and evening dose to deal with a particularly stressful day. At one point he discusses the possibility that his brain may be causing some of his symptoms, but later in conversation refers again to his imminent "kidney failure." The patient reveals that his brother died 18 months ago from pancreatic cancer. The patient has a history of alcohol abuse 5 years ago.

73. What is the patient's most likely diagnosis?

   A. Adjustment disorder
   B. Somatization disorder
   C. Hypochondriasis
   D. Somatoform disorder
   E. Pain disorder

74. What should be your next step in management?

   A. Admit him to the psychiatric inpatient unit because of his poorly controlled panic attacks and his abuse of clonazepam
   B. Explain to the patient why you would like him to taper the clonazepam and start him on an SSRI and communicate your plan to his PCP
   C. Continue the clonazepam and introduce cognitive behavioral therapy into the treatment regimen
   D. Discontinue the scheduled clonazepam and start lorazepam as needed for anxiety in addition to cognitive-behavioral therapy
   E. Continue the clonazepam and start a noradrenergic antidepressant like bupropion or venlafaxine

End of set

---

75. Your upcoming geriatric community outpatient office rotation will be at a facility known as "Threepoints" because it is situated among three different ethnic-minority neighborhoods. In preparation for this assignment, you review a current textbook about cultural variables in clinical psychiatry. Which one of the following statements is correctly associated with ethnic-minority elderly groups?

   A. Elderly Japanese are expressive about revealing symptoms of depression.
   B. Schizophrenia is underdiagnosed in elderly African Americans.
   C. Elderly Hispanic individuals are high utilizers of mental health care.
   D. Elderly immigrants assimilate more readily than younger immigrants.
   E. Elderly immigrants are more likely to manifest culture-bound syndromes.

The next two questions (items 76 and 77) correspond to the following vignette.

A 27-year-old sexually active postal carrier is being evaluated in your office with signs and symptoms of a moderately severe major depressive disorder. As you begin to discuss the merits of medication treatment, he makes a point to interject that he does not want to take a medication that might interfere with his sex life.

76. Which of the following neurotransmitters is most closely linked to sex drive?

    A. Nitric oxide
    B. Acetylcholine
    C. Dopamine
    D. Serotonin
    E. Norepinephrine

77. Which of the following antidepressants is most likely to maintain this patient's sexual functioning?

    A. Bupropion
    B. Fluoxetine
    C. Paroxetine
    D. Sertraline
    E. Amitriptyline

End of set

---

78. A 46-year-old Gulf War veteran presents to your outpatient office with symptoms of rage attacks, hyperarousal, insomnia, and nightmares of his combat experience. You decide to treat his PTSD with SSRIs, as they have proven beneficial in the treatment of which of the following symptoms of PTSD?

    A. Autonomic hyperarousal
    B. Insomnia
    C. Suspiciousness
    D. Rage attacks
    E. Nightmares

79. A 32-year-old male with a history of localized head injury is visiting his primary care physician's office with his sister. She does not know exactly where he was injured but is able to provide a history of his recent unusual behavior. His sister describes the patient as not acting like himself anymore. Since the accident, he has been impulsive, irresponsible, and without motivation, and he now seems to be a poor decision maker. While in the office, the patient makes inappropriate jokes and frequently uses profanity. On neurological exam, the motor and sensory exams are normal and visual fields are intact. As shown in Figure 79, which area of the patient's brain was most likely affected by the injury?

    A. A
    B. B
    C. C
    D. D
    E. E

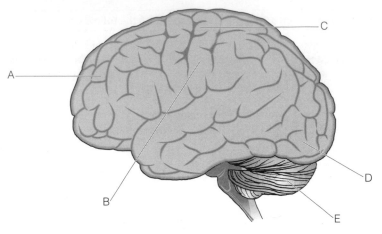

Figure 79

The next four questions (items 80–83) correspond to the following vignette.

A 23-year-old single receptionist has been referred by her gynecologist for psychiatric assessment. She is 8 weeks pregnant and is considering an elective abortion.

80. Which of the following statements is most accurate regarding the psychological effects of an elective abortion?

  A. Most women experience significant psychological sequelae after an elective abortion.
  B. The strongest predictor of poor post-abortion psychological outcome is a history of depression.
  C. Medical or genetic indications for an abortion decrease the likelihood of negative emotional experiences.
  D. A first-trimester decision to abort has the most negative psychological impact.
  E. The rate of PTSD in women who undergo first-trimester abortion is higher than the rate in the general population.

81. An interview of the patient reveals that she has had a significant mood disorder for at least 5 years. She is presently taking valproic acid to control her symptoms. Regarding the special concerns of treating women with bipolar disorder, which of the following statements is true?

  A. Symptoms may recur or worsen premenstrually.
  B. Carbamazepine does not affect contraceptives.
  C. Women with bipolar disorder are at no higher risk for postpartum psychosis.
  D. Valproic acid is not associated with higher rates of fetal anomalies.
  E. Medication levels remain stable across the menstrual cycle.

82. Which one of the following, if true, would be a risk factor for postpartum blues in this patient?

A. Family history of bipolar disorder
B. History of PMDD
C. History of bipolar disorder
D. Previous postpartum psychosis
E. Primiparity

83. The patient decides to continue her pregnancy but stop her mood-stabilizing medication. She does well over the remainder of her pregnancy. Following delivery, which would be the best step to take next in her treatment?

A. Start an antidepressant
B. Electroconvulsive therapy (ECT)
C. Start an antipsychotic
D. Start a mood stabilizer
E. Do nothing

End of set

84. A 38-year-old married administrative assistant is referred by her gynecologist. The patient and her husband have been trying to become pregnant since she stopped using a diaphragm 18 months ago. Which of the following statements is best associated with the psychological factors of infertility?

A. Women tend to be more emotionally affected than their male partners but this effect is short-lived.
B. The demands for sexual performance for men during the fertile portion of the menstrual cycle have few negative effects.
C. Infertile couples typically feel socially supported by their families and peers.
D. Guilt and anger because of past decisions to postpone conception are common problems.
E. It is better to see the two partners individually rather than as a couple.

85. A 53-year-old janitor in your office building is referred for outpatient assessment by her supervisor, who suspects that the patient is a victim of violence. Which of the following statements about female victims of violence is true?

A. Most female victims of sexual assault seek professional help.
B. Rates of sexual abuse are lower in African American women than in the general population.
C. Older women are more likely to be sexually assaulted by strangers.
D. The initial therapeutic approach should be couple, rather than individual, therapy.
E. Female patients presenting with ambiguous physical findings should be evaluated for physical abuse.

86. A 52-year-old single attorney with a history of myocardial infarction and bipolar disorder is seen for her first office visit for lithium maintenance. The patient refuses to tell her primary care physician and cardiologist about her diagnosis of bipolar disorder because she fears the "stigma" of psychiatric illness and is "scared to death" of losing her license to practice law. What would be the best course of action?

    A. Tell her that in keeping her safety in mind, you would be unwilling to treat her unless she allows you to relay her medication list to her other physicians; you would also educate her that legally you are permitted to do so without her consent

    B. Inform the other physicians without the patient's consent, as it is in her best interests, without her knowing that you have done so and have them maintain secrecy on this issue

    C. Encourage the patient to tell her physicians, but reassure her that you would not contact them without her written consent, as it would be illegal and unethical

    D. Enlist a member of her family to disclose the information to her other physicians

    E. Inform her at the end of the interview that because this is an initial consultation, you are not bound by rules of confidentiality and you feel it is necessary to inform her physicians of what she has just disclosed

87. During your primary care treatment team's weekly staff meeting, a nurse practitioner expresses concern that many of the clinic's depressed patients stop taking their prescribed antidepressant medication prematurely. You recently read a research article on this topic. What is the most important variable to accomplish higher adherence to long-term antidepressant therapy?

    A. Planful coping skills training

    B. Favorable attitudes toward antidepressant medication

    C. Involvement in pleasant activities

    D. Increased socialization

    E. Monitoring depressive symptoms

The next five questions (items 88–92) correspond to the following vignette.

A single mother of an 8-year-old boy accompanies her son to your outpatient office. The pair has been referred by the boy's second-grade teacher for assessment of possible attention deficit disorder. During your interview, the boy sits quietly and answers your questions to him succinctly; the mother does most of the talking.

88. Which of the following statements regarding attention deficit hyperactivity disorder (ADHD) is true?

    A. ADHD is limited to childhood years.

    B. The effects of stimulants on ADHD are recently discovered phenomena.

    C. Little scientific literature supports the use of stimulants to treat ADHD.

    D. The use of stimulants to treat children with ADHD is no longer controversial.

    E. There has been a steady increase in the rate of diagnosis of ADHD.

89. After taking a detailed medical and psychiatric history and listening to the mother's observations, it seems the boy may well have ADHD with prominent inattentive symptoms. Which of the following is the best next step?

A. Prescribe methylphenidate twice a day and schedule a follow-up appointment in 3 months
B. Prescribe dextroamphetamine three times a day and instruct the child to keep the mid-day dose in his lunch box to take during recess
C. Prescribe a long-acting stimulant and instruct the mother to not inform the school so there will be no stigma from his teachers
D. Engage the boy's teacher
E. Do nothing and schedule a follow-up visit in 6 months

90. One month later, after baseline ratings of symptoms in the school setting have been made, there is general agreement that a stimulant trial is indicated. Which of the following statements regarding the prescription of stimulants is true?

A. A history of drug abuse is a contraindication to prescribe stimulants.
B. Treated glaucoma is a contraindication to prescribe stimulants.
C. Any cardiovascular disease is a contraindication to prescribe stimulants.
D. Hyperthyroidism is a contraindication to prescribe stimulants.
E. Hypertension is a contraindication to prescribe stimulants.

91. The boy's mother also inquires about the role of play therapy to treat ADHD. Which of the following techniques is most closely associated with play therapy?

A. Emotional catharsis
B. Positive reinforcement
C. Response cost
D. Time-out
E. Token economy

92. Which of the following is the best example of the behavioral technique called "response cost"?

A. Child completes homework and is permitted to play with his or her friends
B. Child pushes classmate on playground and is required to sit alone for 5 minutes
C. Child loses time playing video games for not finishing homework
D. Spanking
E. Child earns stars for completing household chores and can cash them in at the end of the week for a toy

End of set

93. A 76-year-old Navajo man is referred by his daughter, who is concerned that her father is depressed. His wife died 6 months ago, and he seldom leaves the house. Which of the following is the most appropriate first step in the therapy of Native American patients?

A. Indoctrinate the patient to traditional psychotherapy techniques
B. Limit involvement of others
C. Maintain direct eye contact
D. Clarify expectations
E. Minimize genetic influence in regard to psychopharmacology because the patient is elderly

---

The next two questions (items 94 and 95) correspond to the following vignette.

A 36-year-old computer program analyst is required to travel by air frequently. She is seeking outpatient consultation for her fear of flying.

94. Regarding the pharmacokinetics of benzodiazepines, which of the following statements is true?

A. A benzodiazepine's elimination half-life determines how long it accumulates in the body.

B. Benzodiazepine steady-state concentrations are usually achieved over 2 to 3 half-lives of dosing.

C. Benzodiazepines with longer elimination half-lives result in more severe withdrawal symptoms upon discontinuation.

D. Benzodiazepines initially oxidized by hepatic microsomal enzymes have shortened elimination half-lives in the elderly.

E. Benzodiazepines initially conjugated by hepatic microsomal enzymes have prolonged elimination half-lives.

95. Which of the following benzodiazepines is the best to prescribe for this patient for an upcoming cross-country airplane trip for business?

A. Chlordiazepoxide

B. Clonazepam

C. Diazepam

D. Clorazepate

E. Lorazepam

End of set

---

96. A 38-year-old legal assistant is self-referred with symptoms of anxiety, insomnia, and thoughts of suicide. She associates the onset of her symptoms with the termination of a romantic relationship with her employer 2 weeks ago. When you ask her about the relationship, she will only provide evasive answers, implying she fears there could be a breach in confidentiality if she is forthright. Regarding confidentiality in the psychiatrist–patient relationship, what do you tell her?

A. The duty to maintain confidentiality is absolute.

B. Confidentiality ends upon the patient's death.

C. Consent to disclose revealing information is not necessary for scientific reports.

D. Revelation of a past crime warrants breaching confidentiality to law-enforcement authorities.

E. A psychiatrist may release confidential information under legal compulsion.

97. A 33-year-old woman and her 4-year-old son are referred by the son's pediatrician. When you ask the mother about her son, she says, "He never speaks to me . . . he only looks away . . . he either rocks or flaps his hands . . . he stares at lights . . . when I call his name there is no response . . . if I drop a book he shudders . . .". Your initial diagnosis is autism. Which of the following statements regarding autism is correct?

A. Autism is associated with *Streptococcus* infection.

B. Core clinical characteristics include social withdrawal, inflexibility, and impairment in communication.

C. This disorder is limited to children of parents with higher educational and occupational success.

D. Higher rates of developmental and psychiatric disabilities are not observed in family members of autism patients.

E. Few children with autism develop seizures.

98. A 23-year-old single dog groomer is referred for consultation by her psychologist. The patient has been engaged in cognitive-behavioral therapy (CBT) for symptoms of depression, panic disorder, compulsive cleaning, and bulimia the past 18 months but with limited success. Which of the following medications is the best choice to treat this patient's constellation of symptoms?

A. Nortriptyline

B. Phenelzine

C. Sertraline

D. Bupropion

E. Imipramine

The next two questions (items 99 and 100) correspond to the following vignette.

A 53-year-old divorced school teacher is referred for outpatient consultation by another psychiatrist. She has a 20-year history of dysthymic disorder and recurrent depressions with only a limited response to a variety of antidepressants at seemingly adequate doses. When you ask her how she tolerated each of the antidepressants prescribed over the past two decades, she recalls that one in particular made her very sleepy, constipated, and light-headed.

99. Which of the following antidepressants most likely caused these side effects?

A. Bupropion

B. Citalopram

C. Paroxetine

D. Amitriptyline

E. Venlafaxine

100. After further discussion, the patient recalls that she has been treated with amitriptyline, citalopram, paroxetine, and desipramine with little help. Which one of the following antidepressants would be the next logical one to prescribe this patient?

A. Fluoxetine

B. Bupropion

C. Doxepin

D. Imipramine

E. Sertraline

End of set

51.	D	68.	C	85.	E
52.	B	69.	C	86.	A
53.	A	70.	C	87.	B
54.	B	71.	C	88.	E
55.	A	72.	E	89.	D
56.	A	73.	C	90.	E
57.	A	74.	B	91.	A
58.	A	75.	E	92.	C
59.	D	76.	C	93.	D
60.	C	77.	A	94.	A
61.	B	78.	D	95.	E
62.	E	79.	A	96.	E
63.	B	80.	B	97.	B
64.	D	81.	A	98.	C
65.	B	82.	B	99.	D
66.	A	83.	D	100.	B
67.	B	84.	D		

51. | **D.** Donepezil is one of several cholinesterase inhibitors that may be effective in treating the early memory impairment experienced with Alzheimer's disease (AD).

A. Lorazepam, a benzodiazepine anxiolytic, may worsen the memory problems.

B. Risperidone, an antipsychotic, may be helpful in reducing the agitation and psychotic symptoms experienced with dementia but is not presently necessary for this patient.

C. Buspirone, a non-benzodiazepine anxiolytic, may have some efficacy for the anxious patient with dementia, but this patient is not experiencing such symptoms.

E. Sertraline is an SSRI antidepressant. Depression may be manifested as a pseudo-dementia but the MMSE score would likely be higher.

52. | **B.** Rivastigmine, a cholinesterase inhibitor, is helpful in improving the early cognitive and memory deficits experienced with AD. Due to the up-regulation effects of donepezil, its efficacy may diminish; another cholinesterase inhibitor may recapture the positive effect before the disease progresses noticeably.

A. A lower dose of the same medication would not be efficacious.

C. Because the patient does not have any reported psychotic symptoms, risperidone is not necessary.

D. Because the patient does not have any reported depressive symptoms, sertraline is not necessary.

E. Active treatment of cognitive and memory deficits, especially early in the course of AD, can be very helpful to lengthen the patient's period of self-sufficiency.

53. | **A.** Older patients are at increased risk for both EPS and tardive dyskinesia when taking antipsychotic medications. These side effects are less common with atypical antipsychotic agents.

B. Olanzepine is associated with the development of diabetes in all age groups.

C. Quetiapine can cause triglyceride elevation in the elderly.

D. Weight gain can occur in all age groups taking atypical antipsychotic medications.

E. Elderly patients are at increased risk for anticholinergic side effects. The more-sedating typical antipsychotics, such as chlorpromazine and thioridazine, are especially problematic.

54. | **B.** Several controlled trials have suggested that fish oils may be an effective adjunct treatment for bipolar disorder. This supplement might be of benefit to the patient in this case.

A. Some anecdotal evidence suggests that kava may have some anxiolytic properties, but this supplement is not known to affect mood. Reports of hepatotoxicity have caused kava to be banned in some European countries.

C. Valerian has been used as both a sleep agent and an anxiolytic, although currently no objective clinical evidence supports its use. There is no evidence of toxicity or effects on mood with valerian.

D. In randomized, double-blind, placebo-controlled trials, St. John's wort has been shown to have some antidepressant activity and is thus contraindicated in a patient with bipolar disorder. The primary concerns would be elevating the patient's mood into mania or increasing the rate of cycling.

E. Gingko biloba has been reported as being beneficial to memory, although most placebo-controlled trials have failed to show a significant effect. It is not associated with antidepressant or antimanic activity.

55. A. Libido does tend to decrease with age for both men and women.

B. Decreased testosterone levels and increased FSH levels affect men's libido as they age.

C. Decreased estrogen and testosterone levels reduce women's libido.

D. Approximately 80% of all individuals older than 65 years have at least one illness that may affect sexual function.

E. Approximately 25% of men in their seventies and 55% of men older than 80 years report sexual dysfunction.

56. A. SAD often begins early in life with a mean onset at age 15; 35% of the time SAD occurs before age 10.

B. Females are affected with SAD more often than males are.

C. SAD has a lifetime prevalence of 13%, making it the third most common psychiatric disorder after depression and alcohol abuse.

D. The majority of people with SAD suffer from generalized SAD, implying that they fear and avoid most social interaction.

E. Recovery without treatment for SAD is rare.

57. A. SSRIs such as sertraline can be helpful in treating generalized SAD.

B, C, D, E. TCAs such as amitriptyline, imipramine, nortriptyline, and desipramine are not helpful for SAD.

58. A. DLB does account for 15% to 20% of all dementias.

B. Approximately 75% of patients with DLB experience extrapyramidal symptoms.

C. Neuroimaging technologies such as MRI, SPECT, and PET may be useful to differentiate the dementias.

D. Approximately 60% of patients with PD experience minimal cognitive impairment and dementia.

E. The prevalence of AD is 10% for those older than 65 years and 32% for those older than 85 years.

59. **D.** This patient likely has adjustment disorder, acute type, with mixed anxiety and depressed mood. Adjustment disorder is the development of significant emotional or behavioral symptoms due to an identifiable stressor, occurring within 3 months of the stress. An increased risk of suicide is associated with adjustment disorders. Treatment of adjustment disorders typically involves psychotherapy, but treatment with antidepressants is warranted in severe cases.

A. Although the patient is anxious and depressed, the full clinical picture of a major depressive disorder or an anxiety disorder (such as generalized anxiety disorder) is not present.

B. Dysthymia is chronic, low mood that lasts for at least 2 years. This patient has had symptoms for only 3 months.

C. Adjustment disorder is considered chronic if the disturbance lasts for 6 months or longer.

E. In PTSD, a patient exhibits avoidance behaviors, reexperiences the traumatic event, and has symptoms of increased arousal. These symptoms are not indicated in this patient's history.

60. **C.** Curve C illustrates a curvilinear dose response with a therapeutic window; both low and high doses are less effective than midrange doses.

A. Curve A illustrates a curvilinear dose-response but no loss of efficacy at higher doses.

B. Curve B illustrates a linear response.

D. Curve D illustrates a curvilinear dose response with no loss of efficacy at higher doses.

61. **B.** Nortriptyline, a tricyclic antidepressant, is most typically associated with a "therapeutic window" dose-response curve.

A. Desipramine, a tricyclic antidepressant, is more typically associated with a linear dose-response curve.

C. SSRI antidepressant medications such as fluoxetine typically do not have established dose-response curves.

D. SSRIs such as paroxetine do not have established dose-response curves.

E. Risperidone is an antipsychotic, not an antidepressant.

62. **E.** Given that her symptoms developed within 4 weeks of the traumatic event, this patient's symptoms are most consistent with acute stress disorder.

A. If the patient's symptoms persist for longer than 1 month, then her diagnosis will become PTSD.

B. She does not have symptoms of anxiety and depersonalization.

C. There is no indication of the purposeful exaggeration of symptoms or a secondary gain, such as financial reward, that is typical of malingering.

D. Generalized anxiety disorder is a prolonged syndrome of persistent anxiety lasting for more than 6 months.

63. **B.** An SSRI such as sertraline plus the dopaminergic antidepressant bupropion may provide broader neurotransmitter activation and be a relatively safe combination.

A. Fluoxetine and sertraline are both SSRIs and would have limited potentiating effects.

C. The combination of an SSRI, such as sertraline, and an MAOI is always contraindicated. When such agents are used together, a life-threatening serotonergic syndrome can develop.

D. A TCA such as imipramine used cautiously in combination with an MAOI can be a potent antidepressant regimen but is not the safest combination proposed.

E. Lithium can be a valuable potentiator for most all antidepressants but must be used cautiously. Lithium plus the MAOI nardil is not the safest combination proposed.

64. **D.** Diseases that are dermatologic in origin are very rarely associated with the neurovegetative symptoms of depression. Dry skin may be a sign of hypothyroidism, but it would more appropriately fall under the category of endocrine review of symptoms.

A. Common causes of depressive symptoms include hypothyroidism, panhypopituitarism, and adrenal dysfunction. It is important to elicit other signs of these diseases before diagnosing depression.

B. Anemia can be associated with symptoms that mimic depression. Ruling out anemia and other blood diseases is important in the screening process for depression.

C. Patients with neurological diseases such as multiple sclerosis and stroke can appear to be depressed.

E. It is always important to consider infections such as Epstein-Barr virus and HIV before treating someone for depression.

65. **B.** Rapid discontinuation of paroxetine has been associated with a syndrome characterized by paresthesias, headache, nausea, flu-like symptoms, and photophobia.

A. Dry mouth can occur with paroxetine treatment but can also be a side effect of other SSRIs and TCAs.

C. Nausea can be a side effect of paroxetine treatment but is not unique to this medication.

D. Headache is a side effect common to many SSRIs.

E. Delayed ejaculation and decreased libido are side effects common to many SSRIs.

66. | **A.** Short-term memory usually shows a steeper decline and is affected before long-term memory with HIV infection. In particular, attention and learning can be impaired.

B. Psychosis can occur as a result of HIV infection and may signify direct viral effects on the CNS, medication side effects, delirium, opportunistic infection, or a primary psychiatric condition.

C. New psychiatric symptoms may be due to opportunistic CNS infection with fungi, parasites, viruses, or bacteria.

D. Antiretroviral medication side effects can include psychosis, depression, mania, restlessness, agitation, or irritability.

E. Neuropsychological testing of this patient could be beneficial to objectively evaluate the extent of his dysfunction.

67. | **B.** Asking the patient if the voices are telling him to do anything is the single most important follow-up question. Command auditory hallucinations can be very disturbing to patients. If the patient is hearing commands, then inquiring whether he feels compelled to follow the commands would be the next question to ask with regard to the patient's immediate safety.

A. Asking whether the voice is male or female may help elicit discussion, but assessing the patient's immediate safety is much more important.

C. Inquiring about the patient's feelings may elicit further discussion, but it less important than asking about command hallucinations.

D. Referral to a mental health professional may be appropriate in this case, but determining the patient's immediate dangerousness to himself or to others is the primary concern.

E. While medication compliance may be questionable in a patient with new-onset hallucinations, assessment of his safety should be the primary concern.

68. | **C.** This patient's symptoms are suggestive of a transvestic fetishism. The most appropriate step is to explore the reasons he finds his behavior disturbing. The self-loathing typically found with this disorder usually will respond to psychotherapy.

A. Sexual reassignment surgery is sometimes used in the treatment of gender identity disorder, not transvestic fetishism.

B. Exogenous progesterone may be used to treat some paraphilias but would probably not be appropriate to treat someone with transvestic fetishism, as libido and other areas of sexual function are likely to be affected as well.

D. The prevalence of this disorder is unknown. It would be dishonest and misleading to try to comfort the patient by trying to tell him that "many men" participate in this behavior.

E. Disclosing this behavior to his spouse may or may not improve his self-image or may just cause interpersonal conflict. The more immediate concern here is to address why the *patient* feels disgusted by his behavior.

69. **C. The male to female ratio for depression is 1:1 in childhood but during adolescence approaches the 1:2 ratio associated with adulthood.**

A. The prevalence of depression is approximately 2% in children.

B. The prevalence of depression in adolescents ranges from 4% to 8%, approaching the higher prevalence rate as the age group approaches adulthood.

D. SSRIs are the antidepressants of choice for children and adolescents. Despite their widespread use, relatively few controlled studies have examined the effects of these drugs in younger patients.

E. As in adults, antidepressants should be continued in children at the same dose to maintain remission unless significant dose-related side effects arise. Treatment should continue at the successful dose for at least 6 to 12 months.

70. **C. Modafinil is indicated to improve wakefulness in patients with excessive daytime sleepiness.**

A. Sertraline is an antidepressant. Because there are no symptoms except low energy to indicate a depression in this case, it would not be indicated in this patient.

B. Ziprasidone is an atypical antipsychotic. Because there are no symptoms of psychosis in this case, it would not be indicated in this patient.

D. Carbamazepine is an anticonvulsant also used as a mood stabilizer in bipolar disorder. Because there are neither seizures nor mood symptoms in this case, it would not be indicated in this patient.

E. Rivastigmine is an acetylcholinesterase inhibitor used in patients with dementia.

71. **C. Modafinil binds to dopamine reuptake sites, causing an increase in extracellular dopamine but not an increase in its release.**

A. Modafinil does not block serotonin reuptake; this effect occurs with SSRI antidepressants.

B. Modafinil does not block dopamine receptors; this effect occurs with antipsychotics.

D. Modafinil does not affect GABA; this effect occurs with anxiolytics.

E. Modafinil does not stabilize neuronal membranes; this effect occurs with anticonvulsants.

72. **E. Modafinil can cause both hypertension and hypotension.**

A. No specific symptoms of withdrawal are typically observed upon stopping modafinil, although it is likely that the patient's sleepiness will return.

B. Caution should be used when prescribing any medication that affects the CNS.

C. As a stimulant, modafinil can precipitate symptoms of mania, psychosis, and anxiety but is not expected to produce depression.

D. Modafinil can both induce and suppress various cytochrome P-450 isoenzymes.

73. C. This patient meets the criteria for a diagnosis of hypochondriasis, a specific type of somatoform disorder in which there is a preoccupation with the idea that one has a serious disease based on one's misinterpretation of bodily symptoms. The preoccupation persists despite appropriate medical evaluation and reassurance. The belief does not have a delusional intensity (as in delusional disorder, somatic type). The duration of the disturbance is at least 6 months. With this patient's history, it is apparent that the preoccupation with his health is the cause of the panic attacks and depressive symptoms. The likelihood of an underlying or secondary depression or anxiety disorder should always be considered with hypochondriasis. Physical disease must be excluded as well.

A. Although the patient suffered from the loss of his brother 18 months ago, an adjustment disorder as defined in DSM-IV occurs within 3 months of a traumatic or stressful event and resolves within 6 months of the onset of the stressor (assuming that the stressor and its consequences have ended).

B. This patient does not meet the criteria for a diagnosis of somatization disorder, which requires that a person have four distinct complaints of pain, two non-pain gastrointestinal symptoms, and one pseudo-neurological symptom, all beginning before age 30 and occurring over a period of several years; these symptoms must not be fully explained by a medical condition after appropriate investigation to warrant this diagnosis.

D. Enough information is presented for the diagnosis of a specific type of somatoform disorder, hypochondriasis, which causes anxiety due to the preoccupation with disease that is present most of the time.

E. Pain is not this patient's main complaint. What seems to be of most concern to him is the anxiety related to the fear of having serious disease.

74. B. Treatment is most effective when there is collaboration between a PCP who continues regular appointments and a consulting psychiatrist who focuses on coping skills and treats symptoms of anxiety, depression, or psychosocial distress. First-line treatment for hypochondriasis is an SSRI, which would target both depression and anxiety. Because some SSRIs can worsen anxiety early in treatment, it is important to start with the smallest possible dose and increase the dose slowly. Most likely, the dose will have to be increased to the higher range to adequately treat the patient's panic attacks. Some studies have shown that individuals with a history of alcohol abuse are more vulnerable to abusing benzodiazepines, as in this patient.

A. Although the patient does have recurrent thoughts of death, he does not currently have active suicidal thoughts and is not in imminent danger of hurting himself or others. Thus hospitalization is not warranted.

C. It is best to discontinue the benzodiazepine, clonazepam, because of the patient's higher risk of substance abuse.

D. Lorazepam would not be recommended for the same reason as given in the explanation for C. However, CBT can be helpful for treatment of hypochondriasis and to decrease the frequency of panic attacks.

E. SSRIs are first-line therapies because hypochondriasis appears to respond best to a serotonergic agent. If the SSRI is ineffective when administered alone, another medication (e.g., an antidepressant that has a noradrenergic component) can be added as an adjunct therapy. Noradrenergic medications can also be useful for a patient who experiences sexual dysfunction as a side effect of taking an SSRI.

75. **E.** Elderly individuals more often manifest culture-bound syndromes, which complicates making an accurate diagnosis.

A. Japanese are socialized to behave in a deferential manner, which may result in inhibition about revealing emotional symptoms to an authority figure such as a psychiatrist.

B. Both schizophrenia and dementia are overdiagnosed in elderly African Americans.

C. Both Hispanic and Asian elderly persons underuse mental health services.

D. Migration at a later stage of life is often marked by more difficulty acculturating.

76. **C.** Sex drive, or libido, is the first stage of sexual response. This dopaminergic function is mediated by the mesolimbic region of the brain.

A. Nitric oxide is a chemical messenger that controls erections in the penis, which is a major component of the second stage of the sexual response cycle.

B. Acetylcholine is an autonomic parasympathetic neurotransmitter also involved in the second stage of the sexual response cycle, resulting in erections for men and lubrication and swelling for women.

D. Serotonin exerts inhibitory actions on orgasm, the third stage of the sexual response cycle.

E. Norepinephrine is a noradrenergic sympathetic neurotransmitter facilitating ejaculation and orgasm in the third stage of sexual response.

77. **A.** Bupropion is a dopaminergic antidepressant. Not only is it least likely to interfere with this patient's sexual functioning, but it may actually enhance it.

B. Fluoxetine, an SSRI, may result in inhibitory actions on orgasm.

C. Paroxetine, an SSRI, may result in inhibitory actions on orgasm.

D. Sertraline, an SSRI, may result in inhibitory actions on orgasm.

E. Amitryptyline, a TCA, has both serotonergic and anticholinergic properties, potentially causing inhibition of both orgasm and erection.

78. **D.** Rage, impulsivity, suicidality, depressed mood, panic symptoms, and obsessional thinking associated with PTSD may be helped by SSRIs.

A. Autonomic hyperarousal may be helped by beta blockers and benzodiazepines, which should be used cautiously in patients with PTSD because of the frequent concomitant alcohol and substance abuse.

B. Insomnia may also be helped by benzodiazepines, other sedative-hypnotics, and clonidine.

C. Antipsychotics are not routinely used for PTSD but may prove helpful in low doses for paranoia and suspiciousness.

E. Clonidine, a presynaptic α-adrenergic agonist, may be helpful for traumatic nightmares.

79. **A.** The presentation is similar to the case of Phineas Gage, a laborer whose left frontal lobe was impaled by an iron bar after an accidental explosion. The classic frontal lobe syndrome is characterized by poor judgment, disinhibition, irresponsibility, and social inappropriateness.

B. The postcentral gyrus is associated with sensory function; an injury to this area would result in abnormal sensory findings on exam. If the motor sensory cortices had been affected, then abnormal neurological findings would be present.

C. The precentral gyrus is associated with motor function; an injury to this area would result in abnormal motor findings on exam.

D. The patient's visual fields are intact, indicating that the occipital lobe is unaffected.

E. A lesion in the cerebellum would cause difficulty with balance and coordination.

80. **B.** A history of depression is the strongest predictor of poor post-abortion psychological outcome.

A. Of course, some women experience significant distress after an elective abortion, but most do not.

C. Medical or genetic indications for an abortion increase the likelihood of negative emotional experiences.

D. Mid-trimester abortion increases the likelihood of negative emotional experiences.

E. The rate of PTSD in first-trimester post-abortion women is lower than the rate in a general age-related female population.

81. **A.** Mood symptoms frequently recur or worsen premenstrually.

B. Carbamazepine, an anticonvulsant used as a mood stabilizer for bipolar patients, may render oral contraceptives ineffective.

C. Women with bipolar disorder are at higher risk for postpartum psychosis.

D. Mood-stabilizing agents such as carbamazepine, valproic acid, and lithium, especially if taken in the first trimester of pregnancy, are associated with higher rates of fetal anomalies.

E. Medication levels fluctuate across the menstrual cycle.

82. **B. PMDD is associated with a higher risk for postpartum blues.**

A. A family history of bipolar disorder is a risk factor for postpartum psychosis but not postpartum blues.

C. A history of bipolar disorder confers a 35% risk for postpartum psychosis.

D. A previous postpartum psychosis is associated with a 30% risk of recurrence following delivery.

E. Primaparity increases the risk of postpartum psychosis but not necessarily postpartum blues.

83. **D. This patient is at significant risk for postpartum psychosis. Initiation of a mood-stabilizing agent in her third trimester or immediately after delivery can reduce the rate of relapse.**

A. An antidepressant alone would be contraindicated in a bipolar patient because it may cause rapid mood cycling or mania.

B. ECT is used as an alternative for patients who do not respond to medications.

C. The patient is not presently psychotic, so an antipsychotic is not indicated.

E. Considering the patient's history, prophylactic pharmacologic treatment is indicated. Patients with postpartum psychosis are at risk for child abuse, infanticide, and suicide.

84. **D. Women who have purposely postponed childbearing not uncommonly experience guilt and anger for being unsuccessful at achieving pregnancy.**

A. Women tend to be more emotionally affected by infertility than men, and this condition persists after years of treatment.

B. Sexual performance for men during fertile periods can become an issue, especially if they have anxious personalities.

C. Infertile couples typically become socially isolated from their families and friends to avoid painful questions and preoccupations with child rearing.

E. Even if one member of the infertile couple is more psychiatrically distressed, it is more helpful to see both partners as a couple for several sessions.

85. **E. Female patients with ambiguous physical findings should be queried privately about sexual and physical abuse.**

A. Only 1 in 10 female victims of sexual assault seeks treatment.

B. Approximately 20% of all women, 15% of female college students, and 12% of adolescent girls have experienced sexual abuse or assault. These rates are higher for African American women.

C. Although sexual assault affects women of all ages, older women are more likely to be sexually assaulted by marital or ex-marital partners.

D. Individual therapy is indicated first in suspected sexual or physical abuse, as couple therapy is likely to cause defensive behaviors.

86. **A.** Confidentiality can be waived within the clinical treatment circle. Therefore, one does not need to obtain specific consent to discuss information with other members treating the patient, or with supervisors or consultants. This is true even under the new HIPAA regulations. The patient should be told that treatment cannot continue if she is not agreeable to you communicating critical health data to her other treating physicians.

B. This plan does not fall under beneficence, disregards patient autonomy, and would be unethical.

C. On the contrary, *not* informing her other physicians could be extremely dangerous for the patient's health. Other examples that would not require written consent would be in emergencies, when treating a minor, or if the patient is incompetent.

D. The patient's consent is needed to share information with his or her family, with similar exceptions as stated above.

E. A consultant doing an initial evaluation does not have a relationship with the patient and would be able to relay relevant findings and history to the physician who requested the consultation. The patient should be informed of this possibility at the beginning of the consultation. In this instance, the patient was not first educated about this fact.

87. **B.** Long-term adherence to antidepressant therapy is a frequent problem in a primary care practice. Active intervention by the treatment team has consistently been found to be helpful. More recent studies have found that instillation of a favorable attitude toward antidepressant treatment by the professional staff as well as confidence in the side-effects management are the most significant variables to promote adherence.

A. Planful coping does not affect medication adherence.

C. Involvement in pleasant activities does not significantly affect medication adherence.

D. Increased socialization does not significantly affect medication adherence.

E. The self-management activities of checking for depressive symptoms do not significantly improve medication adherence.

88. **E.** Over the past two decades, there has been a steady increase in the diagnosis of ADHD.

A. ADHD is now known to persist into adolescence and adulthood, and adults are increasingly being treated for this disorder.

B. The effects of stimulants on the disruptive behavior of ADHD were discovered in 1937.

C. Studies of the short-term benefits of stimulants on the symptoms of ADHD constitute perhaps the largest body of scientific literature for any childhood psychiatric disorder.

D. The use of stimulants to treat children remains controversial, particularly among the lay media.

89. **D.** Teacher ratings of ADHD symptoms using age and sex-normed instruments should be obtained at baseline and after treatment has begun.

A. Although a stimulant such as methylphenidate may well be indicated eventually, baseline target symptoms in school should be identified first.

B. Baseline target symptoms in the school setting should be identified and arrangements made for school personnel to provide supervision for in-school doses of medications.

C. Engagement of appropriate school staff (e.g., teachers, nurses, coaches) is in the best interest of the child.

E. Minimally, formal assessment of the child's symptoms in school should be documented and monitored.

90. **E.** Untreated hypertension, concomitant use of MAOIs, and active psychosis are contraindications to stimulant use.

A. Stimulants are not contraindicated but should be used cautiously if there is a history of drug abuse. If a member of the household has a history of stimulant abuse, steps should be taken to ensure that the medications are not abused.

B. Untreated glaucoma is a contraindication to stimulant use.

C. Untreated cardiovascular disease is a contraindication to stimulant use.

D. Untreated hyperthyroidism is a contraindication to stimulant use.

91. **A.** Play therapy is a psychological intervention designed to evaluate and change a child's emotional status through catharsis. It has little documented efficacy in the treatment of ADHD.

B. Positive reinforcement provides rewards contingent on the child's performance; it is more closely associated with behavior therapy.

C. Response cost includes withdrawing rewards or privileges contingent on the performance of problem behavior; it is more closely associated with behavior therapy.

D. Time-out involves removing access to positive reinforcement contingent on problem behavior.

E. Token economy includes earning rewards that may be cashed in; it is associated with behavior therapy.

92. | **C.** Losing playtime for not finishing homework is an example of the behavioral technique known as response cost.

A. Being allowed to play after completing homework is an example of positive reinforcement.

B. Having to sit alone after pushing is an example of the time-out technique.

D. Spanking, although in the realm of response cost, is more appropriately termed aversive conditioning.

E. Earning tokens for a grander reward is an example of a token economy.

93. | **D.** As with all cultural subgroups, some Native American patients do not know what is expected of them when seeing a mental health professional.

A. The therapist must be mindful to be sensitive and flexible to the cultural influences that a Native American patient brings to the therapy situation.

B. Consultation with resources such as the tribe, Indian Health Services, family members, and traditional healers can all be of assistance.

C. Direct eye contact may be seen as a sign of disrespect by some Native Americans and may generate anxiety.

E. As with other ethnic groups, there may be variations in the response to the dosages of psychotropic medications compared to the standard doses prescribed to Caucasians. The patient's age also affects medication prescribing.

94. | **A.** A benzodiazepine's elimination half-life determines how long it accumulates in the blood and brain.

B. Benzodiazepine steady-state concentrations are usually achieved over 4 to 5 half-lives of dosing.

C. Benzodiazepines with longer elimination half-lives result in less severe withdrawal symptoms upon discontinuation.

D. Benzodiazepines metabolized by oxidation have longer elimination half-lives, so they should be prescribed cautiously in the elderly and patients with liver disease.

E. Benzodiazepines metabolized by conjugation have shorter elimination half-lives.

95. E. The duration of a benzodiazepine's effect following a single dose is primarily related to its distribution half-life rather than its elimination half-life. A short-acting benzodiazepine such as lorazepam would be the best choice from this list because of its relatively intermediate onset (1 to 6 hours) and distribution times and its short elimination half-life (10 to 20 hours).

A. Chlordiazepoxide has a slow distribution time and long elimination half-life (30 to 200 hours).

B. Clonazepam has a longer elimination half-life (18 to 50 hours).

C. Diazepam has very fast onset (0.5 to 2 hours) and distribution times, but a long elimination half-life (30 to 200 hours).

D. Chlorazepate has fast onset and distribution times, but a long elimination half-life (30 to 200 hours).

96. E. Proper legal compulsion and patient authorization are the two mainstays of disclosing confidential information.

A. The duty to maintain confidentiality is not absolute. Exceptions to confidentiality include the duty to warn and evidence of child abuse.

B. Ethically, confidences survive the patient's death.

C. If a patient's identity cannot be disguised, consent must be obtained before publication.

D. Typically, revelation of a past crime does not warrant breaching confidentiality unless it is recent, particularly heinous, and likely to be repeated.

97. B. Social withdrawal, inflexibility, and communication impairment are core clinical characteristics of autism.

A. *Streptococcus* infection is associated with the abrupt onset of tics in children.

C. There is no special social class issue that distinguishes parents of children with autism.

D. Genetic research of autism shows associations with other developmental and psychiatric disabilities in family members.

E. As many as 25% of persons with autism develop seizures.

98. C. The SSRI sertraline is the best choice among the medications listed, because SSRIs are efficacious in treating depression, panic disorder, OCD, and bulimia.

A. The TCA nortriptyline is not helpful in treating OCD.

B. The MAOI phenelzine is not helpful in treating OCD.

D. The antidepressant bupropion is not helpful in treating panic disorder, OCD, or bulimia.

E. The TCA imipramine is not helpful in treating OCD.

99. **D.** Amitriptyline is a TCA. Its potency for blocking histamine, acetylcholine, and α-adrenergic receptors, resulting in sedation, constipation, and lightheadedness, respectively, is very high.

A. Bupropion has essentially no histamine-, acetylcholine-, and α-adrenergic-blocking properties.

B. Citalopram has minimal histamine-blocking properties and no effect on acetylcholine or adrenergic neurotransmitters.

C. Paroxetine has minimal anticholinergic properties but no histamine- or α-adrenergic-blocking properties.

E. Venlafaxine has no histamine-, acetylcholine-, or α-adrenergic-blocking properties.

100. **B.** Bupropion, a dopamine-enhancing antidepressant, would be the next logical choice from this group. The patient reports a poor response to serotonergic and noradrenergic antidepressants in the past.

A. Fluoxetine is an SSRI, as are citalopram and paroxetine, which have not helped the patient in the past.

C. Doxepin is a TCA much like amitriptyline with serotonergic and noradrenergic properties that have not particularly helped the patient in the past. It also has a higher propensity for histamine, acetylcholine, and α-adrenergic blocking-properties that were problems for this patient in her earlier treatment.

D. Imipramine is another TCA similar to amitriptyline and doxepin in efficacy and side effects.

E. Sertraline is an SSRI similar to citalopram and paroxetine, which evidently were not helpful to the patient in the past.

Setting 3: Inpatient Facilities

You have general admitting privileges to the hospital. You may see patients in the critical care unit, the pediatrics unit, the maternity unit, or recovery room. You may also be called to see patients in the psychiatric unit. A short-stay unit serves patients who are undergoing same-day operations or who are being held for observation. There are adjacent nursing home/extended-care facilities and a detoxification unit where you may see patients.

101. An 83-year-old female with a history of aortic valve stenosis and hypertension was admitted to the hospital 2 weeks ago for worsening dyspnea. Her outpatient medications included citalopram and alprazolam. She denied any alcohol use. She has never abused her anxiolytic medication and has been on the same dose for the past 14 years. Her alprazolam was ordered at half her usual outpatient dose on admission. For the past 10 days she has been "seeing people" around her bed at night. She is also very anxious about the aortic valve replacement scheduled later in the week. The patient has a nearly perfect score on her MMSE and has no previous diagnosis of dementia. She has not shown any confusion or any change in her sleep-wake cycle. Which of the following is most likely the source of her visual hallucinations?

A. Dementia of the Alzheimer's type
B. Schizophrenia
C. Schizoaffective disorder
D. Delirium secondary to general medical condition
E. Benzodiazepine withdrawal

102. A 51-year-old female with a history of coronary artery disease and previous myocardial infarction is admitted for chest pain. Her cardiologist requests that she be evaluated by the consultation service for complaints of chronic chest pain, pain in both of her lower extremities, migraine headaches, and abdominal pain. The abdominal pain is accompanied by nausea and vomiting. On admission she also expresses concern about new-onset "seizures." Her cardiologist, who reveals that this is her tenth admission in the past year, states that an EEG was normal. During these episodes she has tremors in all four extremities, remains conscious for the duration of the episode, and does not have postictal confusion. She had a hysterectomy for "excessive bleeding" when she was 28 years old. Her cardiologist asks for advice about "setting rules" due to the fact that every week she either calls him at home complaining of "10 out of 10 chest pain" or drops by his office unexpectedly for an emergency visit. What is her most likely diagnosis?

A. Pain disorder
B. Undifferentiated somatoform disorder
C. Somatization disorder
D. Hypochondriasis
E. Conversion disorder

103. A 19-year-old Asian honors college student is admitted to the inpatient psychiatric service. She exhibits pressured speech, admits to having racing thoughts, and appears unable to sit still. Her family relates that she has not slept for more than 2 or 3 hours each night since she came home 1 week ago for spring break. Despite being difficult to direct during interview, she is fairly compliant with staff requests but is suspicious of the other patients. When one male patient walks by, she states that she can "feel evil" emanating from him. She also believes that she has special healing powers. Her family reveals that she was started on isoniazid 2 weeks ago for having a positive skin test for tuberculosis. Her urine drug screen is negative, and the patient has no family history of bipolar disorder. What is her most likely diagnosis?

A. Major depressive disorder
B. Bipolar disorder, type I
C. Substance-induced mood disorder
D. Schizophrenia
E. Hypomania

104. A consultation is requested for a surgery patient for a "change in mental status." The patient is a 77-year-old female who is 2 days status post surgery for hip fracture repair. Her chart indicates no prior psychiatric history. The patient's vital signs are as follows: temperature 101.8°F, heart rate 97, respiratory rate 26, blood pressure 156/97. Her current medications include Colace, glucophage, lisinopril, propranolol, and IV meperidine for pain. Upon examination, the patient is disoriented to location, day, date, and year. She is agitated, pulling at soft restraints and yelling, "They're all out to get me! I can see them standing in the shadows!" What is the most likely diagnosis for this patient?

    A. Schizophrenia
    B. Delusional disorder
    C. Delirium
    D. Dementia
    E. Brief psychotic disorder

The next two questions (items 105 and 106) correspond to the following vignette.

A disheveled, middle-aged man has been admitted to the inpatient teaching service for assessment of suicidal ideation to jump in front of a bus. He has a very strong odor of alcohol and various neurological signs on physical exam, including ophthalmoplegia, weakness, confusion, and a staggering gait.

105. This history and findings are most likely related to which of the following vitamin deficiencies?

    A. Vitamin B_{12}
    B. Vitamin A
    C. Ascorbic acid
    D. Niacin
    E. Thiamine

106. The ophthalmoplegia associated with this patient's Wernicke's encephalopathy is related to which of the following?

    A. External strabismus
    B. Conjugate gaze
    C. Ptosis
    D. Sixth cranial nerve palsy
    E. Seventh cranial nerve palsy

End of set

107. As a member of the hospital's professional staff, you are asked to participate on the pharmacy committee. Which of the following medications is a nonstimulant medication approved by the FDA to treat ADHD?

    A. Citalopram
    B. Amitriptyline
    C. Atomoxetine
    D. Methylphenidate
    E. Dextroamphetamine

The next two questions (items 108 and 109) correspond to the following vignette.

A 36-year-old graduate student is hospitalized for a recurrence of his bipolar disorder. This is his fourth hospitalization for manic symptoms during the past 10 months.

108. Which of the following statements is true about the symptom phenomenology of bipolar disorder?

    A. Bipolar patients are symptomatically ill approximately 10% of the time.
    B. Approximately 80% of bipolar patients relapse within 5 years.
    C. Bipolar patients do best with pharmacologic treatment alone.
    D. Manic symptoms typically initiate rapid cycling.
    E. Duration of episodes is approximately 1.5 months for depression and 3 months for mania.

109. Regarding the socioeconomic costs of bipolar disorder, which of the following statements is true?

    A. Bipolar disorder is among the top 10 disabling disorders as measured by disability-adjusted life-years.
    B. Hospitalization costs outweigh bipolar disorder's indirect costs to society and families.
    C. Subsyndromal symptoms cause less social disruption than acute phases.
    D. Despite the nature of their illness, bipolar patients tend to remain married.
    E. There is little correlation between relapse and psychosocial functioning.

End of set

The next three questions (items 110, 111, and 112) correspond to the following vignette.

A 23-year-old single college student was very distraught over her break-up with her boyfriend of 2 weeks. She was admitted to the hospital because she was cutting her forearms and threatening to overdose on her prescribed medications. Her symptoms have now stabilized, and the treatment team is developing a plan for her follow-up care.

110. Which of the following is the most appropriate antidepressant to prescribe to this patient?

A. Fluoxetine
B. Phenelzine
C. Parnate
D. Amitriptyline
E. Imipramine

111. The team's faculty supervisor suggests a treatment trial with venlafaxine. Before prescribing venlafaxine, which particular vital sign should be assessed and documented?

A. Weight
B. Blood pressure
C. Temperature
D. Respiration
E. Pulse

112. Which of the following types of psychotherapy is best indicated in a patient with a borderline personality disorder (BPD) and the symptoms described for this patient?

A. Psychoanalysis
B. Psychodynamic psychotherapy
C. Cognitive therapy
D. Behavioral therapy
E. Dialectical behavior therapy (DBT)

End of set

---

113. A 20-year-old Caucasian male with a history of gang involvement and imprisonment for aggravated assault is transferred from the jail psychiatric inpatient unit for evaluation of suicidal ideation. When asked about his history of violence, he states that he cannot remember the details of the assault. He recounts other similar episodes of "blanking out" and being unable to recall past events. He admits that he was out "partying" with friends immediately before the assault took place. Which of the following conditions should be considered in the DSM-IV Axis II differential diagnosis?

A. Antisocial personality disorder
B. Seizure disorder
C. Substance abuse
D. Dissociative amnesia
E. Malingering

114. A 56-year-old man with chronic alcoholism was admitted to the hospital for pneumonia. Several days into the hospitalization, he developed signs and symptoms of Wernicke's encephalopathy. Although he has since improved, concern remains that he may progress to Korsakoff's syndrome. Which of the following is associated with Korsakoff's syndrome?

A. Reversible short-term memory impairment
B. Impaired sensorium
C. Confabulation
D. Heavy alcohol intake for weeks
E. Structural lesions in the amygdala

115. A 20-year-old homeless man has been admitted directly to the inpatient psychiatric unit. He claims that he cannot remember who he is. He says that he found himself in New York City, but that he cannot recall where he comes from, the circumstances of his trip, or any other information. The only identification he has is a bus ticket from Chicago. Which of the following is the most likely diagnosis?

    A. Dissociative amnesia
    B. Depersonalization disorder
    C. Dissociative identity disorder
    D. Dissociative fugue
    E. Substance-induced amnestic disorder

The next five questions (items 116–120) correspond to the following vignette.

A 26-year-old woman is admitted through the emergency department to the inpatient psychiatric unit. On examination, she demonstrates rapid speech, extreme irritability, and flight of ideas. Although she is too distractible to provide a coherent history, her boyfriend relates that she stopped taking her usual medications nearly 2 months ago.

116. What are the average noncompliance rates among patients with bipolar disorder?

    A. 20% to 30%
    B. 30% to 40%
    C. 40% to 50%
    D. 50% to 60%
    E. 60% to 70%

117. The patient's boyfriend adds that she stopped taking her medication because she did not like the side effects. Which of the following side effects linked to lithium is most commonly associated with noncompliance?

    A. Cognitive dysfunction
    B. Tremor
    C. Weight gain
    D. Acne
    E. Hair loss

118. The patient's boyfriend, a third-year medical student, also relates that she experienced amenorrhea, galactorrhea, and gynecomastia. Which of the following best describes the physiologic mechanism underlying this patient's antipsychotic-induced hyperprolactinemia?

    A. Dopamine-2 (D_2) blockade in the tuberoinfundibular pathway of the brain
    B. D_2 blockade in the mesolimbic area of the brain
    C. D_2 blockade in the mesocortical area of the brain
    D. D_2 blockade in the nigrastriatal pathway
    E. $5HT_{2C}$ receptor affinity

119. After presenting the history of this complicated patient to your faculty supervisor, he quizzes you about the variety of medication-related side effects. Which of the following antipsychotics is most likely to cause hyperprolactinemia in this patient?

A. Risperidone
B. Quetiapine
C. Olanzapine
D. Ziprasidone
E. Haloperidol

120. The patient is also obese. Which of the following atypical antipsychotics is least likely to cause weight gain?

A. Risperidone
B. Quetiapine
C. Olanzapine
D. Ziprasidone
E. Haloperidol

End of set

121. A 28-year-old male with a history of paranoid delusions is brought to the hospital wearing leg shackles and handcuffs. He is accompanied by two armed guards. During a brief break from the examination, one of the guards asks you if you have ever participated in a prisoner execution. Which of the following statements about the involvement of physicians in executions is most consistent with the profession's code of ethics?

A. A physician may assist in an execution by selecting injection sites and starting intravenous lines.
B. A physician may supervise lethal injection personnel.
C. A physician may testify as to medical diagnoses as they relate to the legal assessment of competence for execution.
D. A physician may declare the executed person dead.
E. A physician may witness an execution in a professional capacity.

122. A 32-year-old male is admitted to the inpatient unit for depression with suicidal ideation. He has had two previous trials of antidepressants. The patient says that he has heard about bupropion and is interested in trying it. You counsel him that which of the following statements is true regarding this medication?

A. Its major mechanism of action involves serotonin.
B. The advantage of the sustained-release (SR) formulation is that it is effective when taken once a day and is better tolerated.
C. It is safe for individuals with a history of anorexia but not those with bulimia.
D. The immediate-release formulation can be prescribed for a maximum dose of 300 mg daily.
E. If sexual side effects are a concern, this medication may be better tolerated than an antidepressant that is selective for serotonin.

123. A 53-year-old physician is admitted to the inpatient service with symptoms of weight loss, frequent familiar songs in his head, and visions of friends he knows are not really present. In which region of the brain depicted in Figure 123 (A–E) would you expect a tumor to be present?

   A. A
   B. B
   C. C
   D. D
   E. E

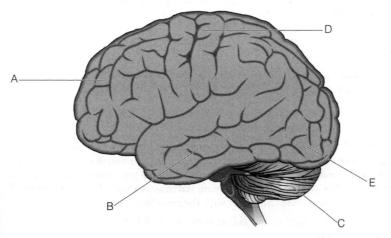

Figure 123

The next three questions (items 124, 125, and 126) correspond to the following vignette.

You have admitted a 22-year-old male with schizophrenia to the inpatient psychiatric unit. He has been started on haloperidol for management of his illness. After taking several doses of the medication, the patient complains of stiffness in his neck and jaw muscles. On exam, cogwheel rigidity is noted in his arms.

124. The patient's symptoms are consistent with a drug effect in which area of the brain depicted in Figure 124 (A–E)?

   A. A
   B. B
   C. C
   D. D
   E. E

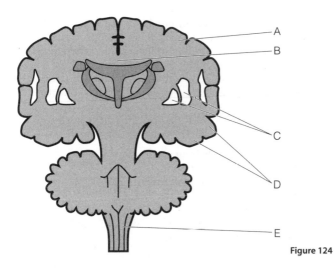

Figure 124

125. Which one of the following medications will provide rapid relief of his symptoms?

A. Benztropine
B. L-Dopa
C. Quetiapine
D. Phenytoin
E. Metoprolol

126. You treat the patient accordingly, and then educate him on the risk of which serious long-term neurological condition associated with haloperidol?

A. Extrapyramidal symptoms (EPS)
B. Parkinson's disease
C. Tardive dyskinesia
D. Huntington's disease
E. Akathisia

End of set

127. A 49-year-old Caucasian male with a history of bipolar disorder, alcohol dependence, and hepatitis C infection is admitted to the medical floor for upper gastrointestinal bleeding, sepsis, and hyponatremia. The patient reports having a depressed mood for the past 9 months after his 20-year-old son committed suicide. Most recently he was on lithium and citalopram, which he stopped taking 3 months ago. He admits to poor sleep, poor appetite, and an increase in crying spells. He denies suicidal ideation but states, "I need to get back on my meds." His labs include the following results: BUN 46, creatinine 1.4, sodium 128, potassium 3.1, AST 138, and ALT 69. Which of the following would be the best step in management regarding his psychiatric medications?

A. Start lithium to prevent a manic episode from occurring
B. Start citalopram due to his depressive symptoms
C. Start lithium and citalopram concurrently to get the patient back on therapeutic doses of his medication as soon as possible
D. Continue to hold his psychiatric medications
E. Start the patient on another mood stabilizer such as valproic acid because the previous medications did not seem to be effective

128. A 29-year-old obese female graduate student is admitted to the inpatient psychiatric unit after an overdose. Her liver enzymes are trending down, and she no longer complains of nausea. She endorses having depression with accompanying anxiety, manifested by restlessness, primary insomnia, and irritability. She meets the criteria for the diagnosis of a recurrent major depression. Although the patient is agreeable to starting a selective serotonin reuptake inhibitor (SSRI), she admits to being wary about antidepressants because she is concerned about their side effects. You counsel her that which of the following statements is true regarding the various medications in this antidepressant class?

A. Paroxetine would be ideal because of its low risk of weight gain.
B. Fluoxetine can be started at 20 mg/day with little risk of increasing her anxiety.
C. Sertraline may cause diarrhea initially, with a decrease in this side effect typically by the second or third week of dosing.
D. Citalopram is purported to have fewer side effects than escitalopram.
E. Sexual dysfunction is a possible side effect of SSRIs but is primarily seen in males and is manifested as erectile and ejaculatory dysfunction.

129. A 33-year-old woman remains in the hospital several days after the cesarean section delivery of a healthy infant boy. You are asked to evaluate the mother because she is experiencing mood lability, tearfulness, and anxiety. Which of the following is her most likely diagnosis?

A. Postpartum psychosis
B. Postpartum depression
C. Postpartum panic disorder
D. Postpartum blues
E. Postpartum obsessive-compulsive disorder (OCD)

130. A 36-year-old married man has been admitted from the emergency center to the inpatient psychiatric unit. Over the past several weeks he has experienced a new onset of psychotic symptoms. On examination, the patient demonstrates choreic movements, dysarthria, and a supranuclear gaze palsy. What is his most likely diagnosis?

   A. Parkinson's disease
   B. Rett's syndrome
   C. Tardive dyskinesia
   D. Sydenham's chorea
   E. Huntington's disease

131. A 68-year-old widower with a history of hypertension and hypothyroidism is being seen in consultation on the inpatient rehabilitation service. He suffered a stroke 2 weeks ago with resultant right-sided hemiplegia and dysarthria. Which of the following statements is true about the psychiatric manifestations of stroke?

   A. Depression occurs in 60% to 80% of stroke patients within 2 years of the initial event.
   B. Stroke lesions producing depression are more commonly found in the right frontal lobe than in the left frontal lobe.
   C. PET reveals bilateral frontal hypometabolism in stroke patients with depression.
   D. Poststroke depression does not typically respond to antidepressant medications.
   E. Mania occurs almost exclusively with lesions of the left hemisphere.

132. A 13-year-old girl with a long-standing history of seizures, excessive nail biting, and recent onset of menses has been admitted to the neurology service. A psychiatric consultation has been requested. Which of the following is true about the risk factors for the development of psychosis in epilepsy?

   A. Seizure focus tends to be right-sided
   B. More frequent in males
   C. Age of onset during latency
   D. Seizure type is often complex-partial
   E. Seizure frequency is increased

The next two questions (items 133 and 134) correspond to the following vignette.

A 29-year-old Marine has been admitted through the Emergency Center to the inpatient unit with symptoms of severe abdominal pain with nausea and vomiting but a soft abdomen, psychosis, and third cranial nerve palsy.

133. What is this patient's most likely diagnosis?

   A. Acute intermittent porphyria
   B. Narcolepsy
   C. Paget's disease
   D. Amaurosis fugax
   E. Pavor nocturnus

134. Which of the following medications might have precipitated the attack described in this vignette?

A. Aspirin
B. Digoxin
C. Penicillin
D. Chloroquinone
E. Tetracycline

End of set

---

135. A 43-year-old married woman with multiple sclerosis (MS) has been admitted to the psychiatric inpatient unit with symptoms of insomnia, trouble concentrating, sadness, and vague thoughts of suicide. Which of the following statements is true about MS?

A. The incidence of MS decreases with latitude.
B. Risk for the development of MS correlates with the latitude at which one lived before age 15.
C. Men are more commonly affected than women.
D. Blacks are more commonly affected than whites.
E. CT scans are more sensitive than MRI for detecting MS plaques.

136. A 26-year-old graduate student with a history of depression has been admitted to the neurology inpatient service for evaluation of persistent headaches. You have been asked to see the patient to evaluate him for mental status changes. The neurologic assessment included an EEG with continuous, focal, polymorphic delta activity with depressed ipsilateral background rhythms. These EEG findings are most consistent with which one of the following diagnoses?

A. Epilepsy
B. Focal brain lesion
C. Early encephalopathy
D. Coma
E. Hepatic encephalopathy

137. A 14-year-old adolescent girl has been admitted to the adolescent psychiatric inpatient unit for evaluation and treatment of anorexia nervosa. The treatment team decides that family therapy is indicated. Which of the following characterizations best describes structural family therapy?

A. Focuses on both the hierarchy of family relationships and the rules of relating that define boundaries within the family
B. Strives to change the repetitive and maladaptive interactional patterns within the family through paradoxical techniques
C. A brief therapy approach that is entirely present-centered
D. Focuses on the understanding of emotions and transference phenomena within the family
E. Relies primarily on object-relations theories

138. A 43-year-old man with a long-standing history of schizophrenia has been hospitalized for the past 10 days after an acute exacerbation of psychotic symptoms and suicidal ideation. The treatment team is meeting to discuss a discharge plan. Which of the following statements about suicide and schizophrenia is true?

A. Approximately 40% of patients with schizophrenia complete suicide.
B. Suicide is more common during middle age.
C. Females with schizophrenia are at higher risk for suicide than are males.
D. Patients with schizophrenia are more likely to complete suicide when their psychosis is under control.
E. Higher education decreases the risk of suicide.

139. A 36-year-old African American male with a history of schizophrenia is admitted to the hospital for pneumonia. He says that he no longer hears voices because he has been stable on clozapine for the past 3 years. Which of the following statements is true regarding this medication?

A. Clozapine differs from other atypical antipsychotics in that it has little effect on the serotonergic system.
B. Because of the 1% to 2% risk for the development of agranulocytosis, monthly monitoring of their white cell counts is mandatory for all individuals taking this medication.
C. Common side effects of clozapine are sedation, excessive salivation, hypotension, hyperthermia, sexual dysfunction, tachycardia, and enuresis.
D. Clozapine is more effective in treating the positive symptoms of schizophrenia than the "typical" antipsychotics such as haloperidol.
E. Clozapine is associated with significant extrapyramidal side effects, including the development of tardive dyskinesia.

140. A 49-year-old married teacher has been admitted to the inpatient psychiatric unit for evaluation and treatment of manic symptoms. Although she has suffered bouts of depression in the past, this occasion is her first psychiatric hospitalization. After treating her with olanzapine and lorazepam for 2 days, the treatment team decides to start her on lithium. Which of the following side effects is most commonly associated with lithium's long-term systemic effects?

A. Weight loss
B. Elevated risk of renal concentrating ability
C. Hyperthyroidism
D. Memory loss
E. Psoriasis

141. A 26-year-old single beautician has been admitted to the inpatient psychiatric unit for treatment of an acute manic episode. Her symptoms include irritability, increased energy, racing thoughts, and rapid speech. She is started on valproic acid and the benzodiazepine clonazepam. Which of the following statements about benzodiazepine treatment is most accurate?

A. High-potency benzodiazepines with short half-lives are less likely to cause physiologic dependence.
B. Low-potency benzodiazepines are associated with treatment-emergent depression.
C. Memory impairment is more commonly associated with high-potency benzodiazepines.
D. The water solubility of benzodiazepines is associated with their effects on memory.
E. The active metabolite of clonazepam is the therapeutic agent.

142. After morning report on the adult inpatient service, the attending psychiatrist asks the first-year residents about the prevalence of psychosis on the unit. Which of the following is the most accurate description of prevalence?

A. The chance of having a negative finding given that no disease is present
B. The proportion of people with a finding or disease in a given population at a given time
C. The chance of having a positive finding given that a disease is present
D. A person without the target condition who has a negative finding
E. The number of new cases of a condition occurring in the population over a specified period of time

---

The next two questions (items 143 and 144) correspond to the following vignette.

A 33-year-old unemployed computer analyst has been readmitted to the inpatient psychiatric unit for treatment of an acute exacerbation of paranoid schizophrenia.

143. Which of the following statements is true about schizophrenia?

A. The onset of symptoms typically occurs earlier in life for women than for men.
B. One in 100 people will develop schizophrenia in their lifetime.
C. Outcome is worse in people with an acute onset of symptoms.
D. Negative symptoms are easier to treat than positive symptoms.
E. The average age of onset of symptoms is 18 years of age.

144. Which of the following is an accurate statement about the evidence-based management of schizophrenia?

A. Chlorpromazine does not improve symptoms any better than placebo.
B. Considerable evidence indicates that polyunsaturated fatty acids reduce the subsequent need for antipsychotic medication in the treatment of schizophrenia.
C. Continuing antipsychotic medication for at least 6 months after an acute episode significantly reduces relapse rates.

D. Social skills training does not reduce relapse rates.

E. Family therapy is likely to improve adherence with antipsychotic medication.

End of set

---

145. A 27-year-old graduate student has been referred for inpatient assessment by his student health center counselor. The student has revealed to his counselor that he has been stalking another student. Which one of the following, if present, would best predict stalking violence in this patient?

A. A major mental disorder

B. Prior sexual intimacy

C. Sobriety

D. Citizenship

E. Threats

The next two questions (items 146 and 147) correspond to the following vignette.

A 46-year-old separated pilot was admitted to the ICU after attempting suicide by overdose with his estranged spouse's medications. His presenting symptoms included hyperreflexia, myoclonus, tremors, confusion, diaphoresis, agitation, and hyperthermia.

146. The patient's symptoms are most consistent with which of the following syndromes?

A. Neuroleptic malignant syndrome (NMS)

B. Lethal catatonia

C. Anticholinergic toxicity

D. Serotonin syndrome

E. Malignant hyperthermia

147. Which of the following medications is most likely causing this patient's syndrome?

A. Chlorpromazine

B. Amitriptyline

C. Haloperidol

D. Alprazolam

E. Paroxetine

End of set

---

148. A 26-year-old lawyer has been admitted to the inpatient substance abuse program for treatment of his cocaine addiction. Which one of the following medications is most likely to dampen his cocaine euphoria?

A. Bupropion

B. Naltrexone

C. Fluoxetine

D. Lorazepam

E. Methylphenidate

149. A 16-year-old high school junior has been admitted to the inpatient substance abuse program. Which of the following statements about alcohol use disorders (AUDs) in adolescents is true?

A. Binge drinking in adolescents usually progresses to alcohol dependence in adulthood.
B. Concurrent use of many substances is the exception rather than the rule.
C. Environmental factors account for a significant amount of AUDs in adolescents.
D. There is less psychiatric co-morbidity in adolescents with AUDs than in adults.
E. Adolescents with early-onset alcoholism are less likely to have familial alcoholism.

150. An 83-year-old retired schoolteacher has been admitted to the inpatient psychiatric unit for evaluation and treatment of her recurrent mood disorder. She also suffers from hypertension, mild congestive heart failure, and emphysema. Which of the following statements about combined drug therapy in the elderly is true?

A. A combination of nefazodone and digoxin increases digoxin serum concentrations.
B. Phenelzine combined with nadolol results in tachycardia.
C. Lithium combined with angiotensin-converting enzyme (ACE) inhibitors lowers lithium levels.
D. Nortriptyline combined with lithium is contraindicated in the elderly.
E. Fluvoxamine combined with theophylline may decrease theophylline plasma concentrations.

Answers and Explanations

Answer Key

101.	E	118.	A	135.	B
102.	C	119.	E	136.	B
103.	C	120.	B	137.	A
104.	C	121.	C	138.	D
105.	E	122.	E	139.	C
106.	D	123.	B	140.	B
107.	C	124.	C	141.	C
108.	B	125.	A	142.	B
109.	A	126.	C	143.	B
110.	A	127.	D	144.	C
111.	B	128.	C	145.	B
112.	E	129.	D	146.	D
113.	A	130.	E	147.	E
114.	C	131.	C	148.	B
115.	D	132.	D	149.	C
116.	E	133.	A	150.	A
117.	C	134.	D		

101. **E.** Physical dependence may occur when benzodiazepines are taken in higher than usual dosages or for prolonged periods of time. Other manifestations of anxiolytic withdrawal include autonomic hyperactivity, tremor, insomnia, nausea, anxiety, and even seizures.

A. Although patients with Alzheimer's dementia can experience hallucinations, this patient's presentation with a nearly perfect score on her MMSE is not indicative of dementia.

B. New-onset schizophrenia is highly unlikely in an 83-year-old.

C. New-onset schizoaffective disorder is unlikely at this patient's age.

D. In a hospitalized elderly individual, delirium should always be considered as part of the differential diagnosis. However, this patient does not show other signs of delirium, such as a change in her sleep-wake cycle, a fluctuating level of consciousness, or agitated confusion.

102. **C.** This patient meets the criteria for a type of somatoform disorder called somatization disorder. A person must have pain in four different body sites or involving four different body functions, two gastrointestinal symptoms (other than pain), one pseudo-neurological symptom (other than pain), and one symptom related to a reproductive organ (other than pain) to be diagnosed with somatization disorder. Some of these symptoms have to be present before age 30 and have persisted for several years. As in this individual, there is often a history of medical and surgical treatments that actually lead to iatrogenic complications. Furthermore, true illness may occur concurrently with somatization disorder, making diagnosis and treatment more complicated.

A, B, D, E. Pain disorder, hypochondriasis, and conversion disorder are types of somatoform disorders. Given the information in this case, the more specific diagnosis of somatization disorder can be made.

103. **C.** This patient has a substance-induced mood disorder, related to isoniazid. Other mental side effects associated with isoniazid include memory impairment and confusion.

A. The patient is not exhibiting symptoms typical of a major depression except diminished sleep.

B. While she meets the criteria for a manic episode with symptoms lasting at least 1 week or requiring hospitalization, the fact that this patient was recently started on isoniazid requires the consideration of a substance-induced mood disorder, as this medication can induce euphoria, agitation, grandiosity, and psychosis.

D. In this young adult, one might consider the possibility of psychotic symptoms related to the onset of schizophrenia, but manic symptoms would generally not be present. Also, her symptoms have not been present for 6 months or longer, which would be necessary to meet the criteria for schizophrenia.

E. The patient's symptoms are typical of mania, not hypomania, and are seemingly caused by exposure to a substance.

104. **C. This is a classic example of delirium.** The diagnosis of an elderly patient with no prior psychiatric history, status post a recent operation, with a sudden change in mental status usually is delirium until proven otherwise. This patient is also febrile and is on an IV narcotic, meperidine, which can cause visual hallucinations, especially in the elderly. The primary treatment of delirium is to correct the underlying organic cause.

A. This patient has no prior psychiatric history, and it is unlikely that she would develop schizophrenia at age 77. Her multiple medical issues make delirium a much more logical choice.

B. The patient is disoriented to location, day, date, and year and having visual hallucinations, none of which would likely occur in a pure delusional disorder.

D. Dementia is a slow, insidious change in cognition and mental status seen over a period of weeks, months, or years. This patient's change in mental status occurred within the last few days, status post an operation, making delirium a more accurate diagnosis.

E. The patient's symptoms are more accurately accounted for by her recent medical history and current medical condition rather than by a nonspecific diagnosis such as a brief psychotic disorder, especially given her advanced age and no prior history of psychiatric illness.

105. **E. Thiamine deficiency is associated with alcoholism and causes Wernicke's encephalopathy.**

A. Vitamin B_{12} deficiency results in pernicious anemia, amblyopia, paresthesias, lower motor weakness, and memory impairment.

B. Vitamin A deficiency results in night blindness, xerophthalmia, and keratomalacia.

C. Ascorbic acid (vitamin C) deficiency results in scurvy. Symptoms of scurvy include lassitude, weakness, irritability, and vague arthralgias.

D. Niacin deficiency results in pellagra. Signs and symptoms of pellagra include glossitis, diarrhea, dermatitis, and mental status changes.

106. **D. A sixth cranial nerve palsy causes the ophthalmoplegia associated with Wernicke's encephalopathy.**

A. A sixth cranial nerve palsy causes internal strabismus.

B. A sixth cranial nerve palsy causes dysconjugate gaze.

C. A third cranial nerve lesion causes ptosis.

E. A seventh cranial nerve palsy causes facial muscle paralysis and loss of taste on the anterior portion of the tongue.

107. **C. Atomoxetine is a clinically effective, FDA-approved nonstimulant useful in treating ADHD. It is a potent inhibitor of presynaptic norepinephrine transporters in the brain.**

A. Citalopram is a serotonergic antidepressant; it is not used for the treatment of ADHD.

B. Amitriptyline is a tricyclic antidepressant; it is not used for the treatment of ADHD.

D. Methylphenidate is an FDA-approved stimulant treatment for ADHD.

E. Dextroamphetamine is an FDA-approved stimulant treatment for ADHD.

108. **B.** Bipolar disorder is both a chronic and a recurrent illness. More than 80% of patients will have a recurrence of depression or mania within 5 years.

A. Bipolar patients are symptomatic 50% of the time, mostly in a depressed phase.

C. Bipolar patients do best with a combination of pharmacologic and psychosocial treatments.

D. Depressed symptoms more typically initiate rapid cycling.

E. Manias tend to be shorter in duration than depressive episodes.

109. **A.** Along with heart disease, cancer, and AIDS, bipolar disorder is a leading disabling illness.

B. Indirect costs such as missed days at work and burden on caregivers far outweigh the costs for direct medical care.

C. Patients with prolonged subsyndromal symptoms have a worse socioeconomic outcome than simple acute-episode counting.

D. Patients with bipolar disorder have a high rate of divorce.

E. Impaired psychosocial functioning causes more stressful events such as the loss of family supports and financial difficulties, which can exacerbate relapses.

110. **A.** Fluoxetine is an SSRI antidepressant that can be helpful in relieving symptoms of anger, depression, and aggressive behavior. It is much safer when overdosed than an MAOI or TCA.

B. Phenelzine is an MAOI; although it is an efficacious antidepressant, it would be contraindicated in this patient because of its high lethality upon overdosing.

C. Parnate, an MAOI, would also be contraindicated.

D. Amitriptyline, a TCA, can be lethal on overdose.

E. Imipramine, a TCA, can be lethal on overdose.

111. **B.** Venlafaxine has a particular side effect of frequently elevating the patient's blood pressure in the range of 5 mm Hg but sometimes produces even higher pressures. This could be problematic in the borderline hypertensive patient.

A. Although there is a potential for weight gain with many psychotropic medications, venlafaxine is not particularly associated with such effects.

C. Temperature elevation is not an expected side effect from venlafaxine.

D. Respiratory changes are not expected side effects from venlafaxine.

E. Any serotonergic agent has the potential to decrease a patient's pulse rate; the nonspecific noradrenergic property of venlafaxine may elevate the heart rate.

112. **E. DBT is a psychotherapeutic strategy specifically helpful for individuals with BPD to decrease suicidal behaviors and mitigate symptomatology.**

A. The uncovering process and ambiguities of psychoanalysis tend to promote regression in the BPD patient, which may result in immature behaviors.

B. Although more directive than psychoanalysis, psychodynamic psychotherapy has a similar theoretical base and tends to be reserved for the higher-functioning BPD patient.

C. Cognitive therapy is merely one element of DBT; both employ collaborative problem solving and a focus on the present.

D. Behavioral therapy is another element of DBT; both use direct reinforcement of behavior.

113. **A. Antisocial personality disorder (like all of the personality disorders) is listed on Axis II. The other listed diagnoses are included in Axis I or III in the DSM-IV format.**

B. A differential diagnosis of dissociative symptoms may include seizure disorder, particularly complex partial seizures (especially those originating in the temporal lobe); head injury; sequelae of electroconvulsive therapy or anesthesia; delirium; or dementia.

C. Substance abuse and withdrawal should always be considered when a patient presents with complaints of memory loss. This is particularly true for this young male, who would be at high risk for alcohol and street drug use.

D. Dissociative amnesia is characterized by an inability to recall important personal data beyond what could be explained by ordinary forgetfulness. It is typically precipitated by an intense psychological trauma or stressor, some threat of harm or death, an intolerable or inescapable life situation, or a morally unacceptable impulse or act.

E. A psychological differential diagnosis of the dissociative disorders includes malingering, particularly if a patient in legal difficulties stands to gain by withholding incriminating information.

114. **C. Korsakoff's syndrome is associated with filling in memory deficits with false information, a condition called confabulation.**

A. Only 20% of patients with Korsakoff's syndrome make a significant recovery.

B. Remarkably, a clear sensorium is typically present.

D. Chronic alcohol abuse for years and nutritional deficiencies cause the syndrome.

E. Postmortem brain studies reveal bilateral lesions in the mamillary bodies rather than in the amygdala.

115. | **D.** Amnesia, unexplained travel, and identity confusion are classic symptoms of dissociative fugue. The treatment approach for dissociative fugue and amnesia includes an adaptational approach in a safe and stable environment. A phasic process with paced retrieval of dissociated information typically works best.

A. Dissociative amnesia is associated with the inability to recall emotionally charged memories; it would not explain this patient's broad symptoms.

B. Depersonalization disorder deals with a sense of detachment from one's body. It would not explain this patient's recent travel, amnesia, or identity confusion.

C. This patient gives no evidence of having multiple personalities, which would be required for a diagnosis of dissociative identity disorder.

E. There is no evidence presented that this patient has abused alcohol or drugs, nor would that explain his recent travel.

116. | **E.** Noncompliance rates among bipolar patients run between 60% and 70%.

A, B, C, D. The 20% to 50% rates are too low in regard to noncompliance among patients with bipolar disorder. After an acute episode resolves, users of lithium take their medication an average of 38% of the days it is prescribed. Only 8% of these patients take the lithium 90% of the days it is prescribed.

117. | **C.** Weight gain is the side effect most commonly related to medication discontinuation.

A. Cognitive dysfunction, including short-term memory and lessened creativity, can occur even with lower or therapeutic lithium levels.

B. Tremor can occur at lower lithium levels but tends to be dose dependent.

D. Acne can occur with lithium use at any age, but especially in adolescent and younger-adult age groups.

E. Hair loss can occur at any lithium level; zinc sometimes helps with this side effect.

118. | **A.** Dopamine-2 (D_2) blockade in the tuberoinfundibular pathway results in loss of normal suppression of prolactin by dopamine.

B. D_2 blockade in the mesolimbic area reduces psychosis.

C. D_2 blockade in the mesocortical area reduces psychosis.

D. D_2 blockade in the nigrastriatal pathway causes extrapyramidal symptoms.

E. $5HT_{2C}$ receptor affinity results in weight gain.

119. | **E.** Haloperidol elevates prolactin levels the most significantly.

A. Risperidone elevates prolactin levels above the normal range but not as severely as haloperidol.

B. Only quetiapine and clozapine are truly prolactin-sparing antipsychotics.

C. Olanzapine produces transient increases in prolactin levels that usually diminish in weeks.

D. Ziprasidone also produces transient increases in prolactin levels.

---

120. **B.** Quetiapine has the lowest affinity of all the atypical antipsychotics for $5HT_{2C}$ receptors; $5HT_{2C}$ blockade is associated with weight gain.

A. Risperidone's affinity for $5HT_{2C}$ receptors is much greater than that of quetiapine but less than that of olanzapine and ziprasidone.

C. Olanzapine's affinity for $5HT_{2C}$ receptors is between that of risperidone and ziprasidone.

D. Ziprasidone has the greatest affinity for $5HT_{2C}$ receptors of the medications listed.

E. Haloperidol is not an atypical antipsychotic. Its affinity for $5HT_{2C}$ receptors is the least of the medications listed.

---

121. **C.** According to the AMA code of ethics, a physician should not be part of a legally authorized execution. A physician may testify regarding medical history, diagnoses of mental state as they relate to competence to stand trial, or competence for execution.

A, B. The prohibitions against involvement in a legally authorized execution include selecting injection sites, starting intravenous lines, and prescribing, administering, or supervising the injection of lethal drugs.

D. A physician may certify death provided that the executed person has been declared dead by someone else.

E. A physician can observe an execution only in a nonprofessional capacity.

---

122. **E.** Bupropion is not commonly associated with sexual side effects; in fact, it is sometimes added to SSRIs to decrease sexual side effects.

A. Bupropion's major mechanism of action is inhibition of norepinephrine and dopamine reuptake.

B. The immediate-release formulation of bupropion may be started at 100 mg twice a day and increased after 3 days to a standard dosing of 100 mg three times a day. The sustained-release formulation of bupropion has allowed the dosing frequency to be decreased to only twice daily. Bupropion SR also has increased tolerability, especially in terms of possibly reducing the frequency of seizures associated with the immediate-release formulation. A third preparation of bupropion (extended release) allows once-daily dosing.

C. A careful eating-disorder history should be obtained before starting a patient on bupropion, as studies have shown an increased risk of seizures in these individuals.

D. The maximum recommended dose of immediate-release bupropion is 150 mg three times daily, for a total of 450 mg/day. Sustained-release bupropion has a maximum recommended dose of 400 mg/day. The risk of seizures is increased significantly when higher dosages are used.

123. | **B.** A patient with temporal lobe tumors may have auditory and visual hallucinations. The hallucinations may recall a previous experience.

A. Frontal lobe tumors typically result in memory disturbance and social inappropriateness.

C. A tumor in the cerebellum would likely cause a problem with balance.

D. A tumor in the somesthetic postcentral gyrus region would cause numbness.

E. A tumor in the occipital lobe would result in a visual deficiency.

124. | **C.** The globus pallidus and putamen are areas of the basal ganglia that receive dopaminergic innervation from the substantia nigra. In combination, these areas are thought to play an important role in movement disorders associated with dopamine-blocking medications.

A. The motor cortex is associated with voluntary movements but not directly with medication-induced movement disorders.

B. The corpus callosum contains fibers that communicate between the right and left hemispheres.

D. Lesions in the temporal lobe may cause behavioral and emotional changes.

E. Lesions in the spinal cord may cause paralysis and paresthesias, but this region is not directly associated with the medication side effects described here.

125. | **A.** This patient is having a dystonic reaction to the haloperidol, also called extrapyramidal symptoms (EPS). Benztropine is an anticholinergic medication that is the best treatment for an acute dystonia. Diphenhydramine is another anticholinergic medication that is typically used for this condition. Both medications may be administered orally or intramuscularly if the patient is having difficulty swallowing.

B. L-Dopa is an accepted treatment for Parkinson's disease, but is not an effective treatment for acute dystonia. Haloperidol is a strong antagonist to the dopamine receptor, and L-Dopa is unlikely to displace the tightly bound haloperidol.

C. Quetiapine is an atypical antipsychotic medication that has a low incidence of EPS, but it would not be an effective acute treatment for a dystonic reaction.

D. Phenytoin is an anticonvulsant that is not an effective treatment for acute dystonias.

E. Metoprolol is a beta blocker that is not an effective treatment for acute dystonias.

126. | **C.** Tardive dyskinesia (TD) is a potentially irreversible involuntary movement disorder associated with the use of dopamine-blocking drugs such as haloperidol. The risk of developing TD and the potential severity are thought to increase with length of treatment and amount of drug exposure. The risk of TD is also thought to be increased in patients who experience dystonic reactions and other EPS as in this case.

A. EPS can include dystonias, akathisia, and cogwheel rigidity. These symptoms may occur during the course of drug exposure, but almost always resolve after the drug is discontinued. While EPS may be a medication side effect, this is not the best answer.

B. EPS can mimic certain features of Parkinson's disease, but these are distinct entities. Development of Parkinson's disease is not associated with use of antipsychotic medications.

D. EPS can mimic certain features of Huntington's disease, but these are distinct entities. Development of Huntington's disease is not associated with use of antipsychotic medications. Patients with Huntington's disease may, over the natural course of their illness, eventually develop psychosis.

E. Akathisia, which is best described as motor restlessness, may cause voluntary movements such as pacing or leg movements. While it may be a side effect experienced during the course of antipsychotic use, it is not the best answer for this question.

127. **D.** In this patient who has hyponatremia and hypokalemia, it would not be prudent to start lithium, as this medication could further disrupt the patient's electrolyte status. His BUN:creatinine ratio is greater than 20:1, indicating that the patient is dehydrated. Lithium, even within the recommended therapeutic range, can cause diabetes insipidus and worsen the dehydration. There is no urgent need to restart the medication. An antidepressant such as citalopram should not be started until the patient is on a therapeutic dose of a mood stabilizer to decrease the risk of precipitating a manic episode. Furthermore, any SSRI can cause (or, in this case, worsen) hyponatremia. The patient should be reassessed periodically during his hospital stay and medications restarted pending resolution of his acute medical problems.

A, B, C. As in the explanation for D, holding this patient's medications is the prudent approach.

E. Valproic acid, which is metabolized in the liver, would not be a good choice in this patient with hepatitis and elevated liver enzymes. Stabilization of the acute physical issues supercedes the need to restart his psychiatric medication.

128. **C.** Like many SSRIs, sertraline can cause gastrointestinal disturbance such as diarrhea, constipation, or abdominal pain. The diarrhea may be quite significant and inconvenient. Patients should be informed that this side effect typically lessens in severity the longer one takes the medication.

A. Paroxetine has been known to cause significant weight gain. In a patient who is already overweight, this agent may not be the SSRI of choice.

B. In a patient who has significant agitation and anxiety in addition to depressed mood, it is a good idea to start fluoxetine at 10 mg/day for several days, then increase the dose to 20 mg/day. Fluoxetine may have an "activating" effect during initial dosing, so starting with a low dose will decrease the risk of increasing the patient's subjective feelings of anxiety and restlessness.

D. Escitalopram is the enantiomer of citalopram and is often better tolerated than the older citalopram.

E. Patients of both genders should be educated about the possible risk of sexual dysfunction with SSRIs, which some studies show to be as high as 70%. This side effect can be manifested as decreased libido, erectile dysfunction, or difficulty with orgasm and ejaculation. Particularly in an individual such as this patient, who views starting medication with some trepidation, it would be prudent to reassure her that many options are available to decrease the severity of this side effect. Some examples would be lowering the dose or adding an adjunct agent such as buspirone or bupropion.

129. **D.** As many as 85% of new mothers experience postpartum blues, which is a temporary condition usually beginning 2 to 4 days after delivery and relenting within 2 weeks.

A. Postpartum psychosis is a serious but relatively rare illness. It is characterized by extreme mood lability, agitation, hallucinations, and delusions.

B. Postpartum depression shows the hallmarks of a major depressive episode and has a prevalence of approximately 10%.

C. Postpartum panic disorder is manifested in much the same way as typical panic disorder and can also occur with or without agoraphobia.

E. Postpartum OCD has gained increased recognition and would be manifested with the expected obsessional and/or compulsive symptoms, none of which is described in this patient.

130. **E.** Huntington's disease is the most likely diagnosis considering the constellation of symptoms.

A. Parkinson's disease is manifested by bradykinesia rather than chorea.

B. Rett's syndrome is manifested by autism, ataxia, and stereotypical hand movements in girls.

C. Tardive dyskinesia is also a choreiform disorder but generally occurs when there has been chronic exposure to dopamine-blocking agents such as the typical antipsychotics. TD would be unlikely in a patient with new-onset psychosis.

D. Sydeham's chorea follows group A streptococcal infections. It can be accompanied by irritability and obsessive-compulsive symptoms rather than psychosis. Psychosis is present in 5% to 15% of patients with Huntington's disease.

131. **C.** PET reveals bilateral frontal hypometabolism in stroke patients with depression.

A. Depression occurs in 30% to 50% of stroke patients. Major depression is not correlated with the severity of disability, whereas minor depression is more closely correlated with the severity of disability.

B. Stroke lesions producing depression are more commonly found in the left frontal lobe.

D. Poststroke depression commonly responds to conventional antidepressants.

E. Mania occurs almost exclusively with lesions of the right hemisphere.

132. **D.** Psychosis is more likely to occur in individuals with a history of complex-partial seizures.

A. The seizure focus tends to be left-sided in those developing psychosis.

B. Psychosis is more frequent in females with seizures.

C. Psychotic symptoms usually start during puberty when they are associated with seizures.

E. Psychosis is associated with a diminished frequency of seizures.

133. **A.** The porphyrias are rare disorders of heme biosynthesis with neurologic, psychiatric, cutaneous, and other organ manifestations. They are caused by autosomal dominant enzyme defects of heme biosynthesis.

B. Narcolepsy is a sleep disorder characterized by excessive daytime somnolence, sleep attacks, cataplexy, and sleep paralysis.

C. Paget's disease is a disorder of local bone remodeling, resulting in pain. It usually develops after age 40.

D. Amaurosis fugax is the symptom of partial or complete transient monocular blindness caused by a transient ischemic attack of the retinal vasculature.

E. Pavor nocturnes, also known as sleep terrors, occurs almost exclusively in children.

134. **D.** Chloroquine is one of many drugs that may precipitate an attack of acute intermittent porphyria. These drugs activate heme biosynthesis.

A, B, C, E. Aspirin, digoxin, penicillin, and tetracycline do not exacerbate acute intermittent porphyria.

135. **B.** The risk for the development of MS is correlated with the latitude at which one lived before age 15.

A. The incidence of MS increases with latitude.

C. Women are more commonly affected by MS than are men.

D. Whites are more commonly affected by MS than are blacks.

E. MRI is more sensitive than CT scan for detecting MS plaques.

136. **B.** Continuous, focal, polymorphic delta activity strongly suggests a focal lesion.

A. Spikes, sharp waves, or spike-wave complexes suggest epilepsy.

C. Early encephalopathy typically causes α-rhythm slowing and generalized theta activity on the EEG.

D. The EEG findings of a coma include lack of normal background and reactivity with continuous, generalized, polymorphic delta activity.

E. Hepatic and other metabolic encephalopathies result in periodic triphasic waves on the EEG.

137. **A.** Structural family therapy focuses on the hierarchy of family relationships and the rules of relating that define the boundaries between the subsystems of the family.

B. Strategic family therapy utilizes paradoxical strategies to change repetitive and maladaptive patterns within the family.

C. Solution-focused family therapy is a brief therapy model focusing only on the present.

D. Psychodynamically oriented family therapy focuses on the understanding of emotions and transference phenomena.

E. Object-relations therapy is a form of psychodynamically oriented therapy emphasizing the importance of projection and projective identification in family relationships.

138. **D.** Patients with schizophrenia are more likely to complete suicide when the psychosis is under control, coincidental with a depressive recovery phase of the illness.

A. Approximately 10% of patients with schizophrenia complete suicide.

B. The majority of suicides in patients with schizophrenia occur in younger patients.

C. Males with schizophrenia—especially younger males—are at a higher risk for suicide.

E. Higher education is associated with increased suicide risk in patients with schizophrenia, perhaps related to a heightened awareness that their lives have become different.

139. **C.** All of these are common side effects of clozapine. Among the atypical antipsychotics, clozapine has very strong anticholinergic effects, compared to quetiapine, risperidone, and olanzapine, which have only mild anticholinergic effects.

A. Clozapine, like other atypical antipsychotics such as olanzapine, risperidone, and quetiapine, has a relatively weak D_2 binding effect combined with a relatively potent serotonergic effect, which accounts for its side-effect profile.

B. Clozapine is a very effective antipsychotic. However, due to its 1% to 2% risk of causing agranulocytosis, a weekly check of the white blood cell count is a must for patients who take this medication; they are often enrolled in "clozapine clinics" for this reason. Sometimes the white cell count can be done every 2 weeks instead of weekly. The risk of agranulocytosis is the main reason why clozapine is used only in treatment-resistant psychosis—that is, after an individual has failed previous trials of antipsychotics.

D. Like other atypical agents, clozapine is more effective at treating the negative, as well as the positive, symptoms of schizophrenia as compared to the typical antipsychotics such as haloperidol.

E. Clozapine appears to carry no risk of TD and is not associated with significant EPS. Researchers propose that atypical agents such as clozapine bind more strongly to D_3, D_4, and D_5 receptors than older antipsychotics such as haloperidol and chlorpromazine. These more recently discovered dopamine receptors are found in the frontal cortex and limbic areas rather than in the striatum, which may account for the decreased risk of EPS and TD.

140. **B.** The long-term effect of lithium on the kidneys is controversial, but the balance of literature suggests an increased risk of impaired renal concentrating ability.

A. As many as 50% of lithium recipients will experience a 5% to 10% weight gain; weight loss is practically unheard of.

C. Hypothyroidism, rather than hyperthyroidism, occurs in lithium recipients at rates of 5% to 35%. This effect is much more common in women.

D. Memory loss—in particular, recall or retrieval—is a dose-related, rather than long-term, effect of lithium.

E. Psoriasis is a rare dermatologic effect of lithium use.

141. **C.** Memory impairment is more commonly associated with high-potency benzodiazepines such as triazolam and lorazepam.

A. High-potency benzodiazepines with short half-lives are more likely to cause physiologic dependence.

B. Treatment-emergent depression is more commonly associated with high-potency benzodiazepines.

D. The lipid solubility, rather than water solubility, of benzodiazepines is associated with impact on memory. Clonazepam has low lipid solubility.

E. There is no active metabolite of clonazepam.

142. **B.** Prevalence is the proportion of people with a finding or disease in a given population at a given time.

A. Specificity is the chance of having a negative finding given that no disease is present.

C. Sensitivity is the chance of having a positive finding given that a disease is present.

D. True negative refers to a person without the target condition who has a negative finding.

E. Incidence is the number of new cases of a condition occurring in a population over a specified period of time.

143. **B.** Schizophrenia is a relatively common illness; one in 100 people will develop schizophrenia in their lifetime.

A. The onset of symptoms for schizophrenia is typically earlier in life for men than for women.

C. Outcome is better in people with an acute onset of schizophrenia symptoms. An insidious onset is generally associated with a worse prognosis.

D. Positive symptoms such as hallucinations, delusions, and ideas of reference are easier to treat than the negative symptoms of apathy, self-neglect, and reduced emotion.

E. The average age of onset for schizophrenia is 25 years.

144. **C.** Continuing antipsychotic medication for at least 6 months after an acute episode reduces relapse rates.

A. Chlorpromazine, the prototypical classic antipsychotic agent, does improve symptoms of schizophrenia better than placebos but has many unpleasant side effects such as sedation, orthostatic hypotension, dry mouth, and EPS at higher doses.

B. Little evidence indicates that polyunsaturated fatty acids reduce the need for antipsychotic medications in schizophrenia.

D. Social skills training compared to medication management alone does reduce relapse rates.

E. Family therapy beyond education is unlikely to improve compliance with antipsychotic medication.

145. **B.** A strong correlation exists between sexual intimacy and stalker violence. This holds true for both male and female stalkers.

A. A major mental illness such as schizophrenia does not positively correlate with stalking violence. Stalkers who are psychotic tend to stalk public figures, whereas those who are not psychotic tend to stalk private individuals.

C. Drug and alcohol abuse are predictors of physical injury during stalking.

D. Several studies found prior criminal convictions to be a predictor of stalker violence, but there is no established correlation with citizenship.

E. Only a moderate predictive relationship exists between threats and stalking violence. This correlation tends to be stronger with stalking private individuals versus public individuals.

146. **D.** The symptoms of hyperreflexia, myoclonus, tremors, confusion, diaphoresis, agitation, and hyperthermia are most consistent with a serotonin syndrome.

A. NMS is typically manifested by severe muscular rigidity, EPS, tachycardia, and hyperthermia.

B. Lethal catatonia has many similarities to NMS.

C. Anticholinergic toxicity results in hot, dry skin, mydriasis, tachycardia, urinary retention, delirium, muscular relaxation, and hyperthermia.

E. Malignant hyperthermia is an inherited disorder whose onset occurs after exposure to specific anesthetic agents that block the neuromuscular junction.

147. E. Paroxetine is an SSRI antidepressant. An overdose with any SSRI could result in a serotonin syndrome.

A. Chlorpromazine is a dopamine receptor-blocking antipsychotic. An overdose with this medication could result in NMS.

B. Amitriptyline is a highly anticholinergic TCA. An overdose with this medication could result in anticholinergic toxicity.

C. An overdose with the antipsychotic haloperidol could result in NMS.

D. Alprazolam is a potent benzodiazepine. An overdose with benzodiazepines results in sedation.

148. B. Naltrexone is an opioid receptor antagonist that might attenuate cocaine euphoria by blocking the endorphins released by cocaine.

A. Bupropion, a dopaminergic antidepressant, could accentuate the effects of cocaine.

C. Fluoxetine, a serotonergic antidepressant, has limited direct effect on cocaine-induced euphoria.

D. Lorazepam, a benzodiazepine, has limited direct effect on cocaine-induced euphoria.

E. Methylphenidate, a dopaminergic stimulant, would enhance the effects of cocaine.

149. C. Environmental factors account for approximately 40% of AUDs in adolescents. They include peer pressure, product advertising, and self-medication for anxiety, depression, and ADHD.

A. Binge drinking in adolescents usually does not progress to alcohol dependence.

B. Concurrent use of many substances such as opiates, marijuana, and cocaine is the rule in adolescents with AUDs.

D. There is more psychiatric co-morbidity in adolescents with AUDs than in adults.

E. Adolescents with early-onset alcoholism are more likely to have familial alcoholism.

150. **A.** Digoxin combined with the antidepressant nefazodone increases digoxin levels by approximately 25%.

B. The beta blocker nadolol combined with the MAOI antidepressant phenelzine results in bradycardia.

C. Lithium combined with ACE inhibitors increases lithium levels.

D. Lithium combined with the TCA nortriptyline can improve response in major depression but should be used cautiously in the elderly.

E. Fluvoxamine, an SSRI antidepressant, inhibits cytochrome P-450 1A2 and, as a result, can increase theophylline concentrations when the two agents are combined.

Questions

Setting 4: Emergency Department

Generally, patients encountered here are seeking urgent care; most are not known to you. A full range of social services is available, including rape crisis intervention, family support, child protective services, domestic violence support, psychiatric services, and security assistance backed up by local police. Complete laboratory and radiology services are available.

The next four questions (items 151–154) correspond to the following vignette.

A 36-year-old Hispanic woman was grocery shopping with her nephew when she experienced a rapid onset of chest pain, diaphoresis, hot flashes, and shortness of breath. She stated that she felt like she was dying. An ambulance was called and transported her to the emergency department (ED), where she was found to be diaphoretic, mildly tachycardic (pulse 106), and hypertensive (142/94). Otherwise, the physical exam was normal. Further testing revealed normal CBC, CMP, cardiac enzymes, and ECG. Urine drug screen was negative. Pregnancy testing was also negative. Within 15 minutes of her arrival to the ED, the patient's vitals had normalized. The patient revealed that she has had several similar but less severe episodes in the past 6 months.

151. What is the most likely diagnosis for this patient?

    A. Delusional disorder, somatic type
    B. Post-traumatic stress disorder (PTSD)
    C. Obsessive-compulsive disorder (OCD)
    D. Panic disorder
    E. Generalized anxiety disorder (GAD)

152. Which of the following specific phobias is strongly associated with this woman's diagnosis?

    A. Apiphobia
    B. Agoraphobia
    C. Claustrophobia
    D. Gynophobia
    E. Hydrophobia

153. Which other lab test is routinely performed on patients with these symptoms and is important for accurate diagnosis?

    A. Thyroid function test
    B. Fasting plasma glucose
    C. Plasma cortisol
    D. Testosterone level
    E. Arterial blood gases

154. Which of the following pharmacologic treatments would most benefit the patient in her acute situation?

    A. Sertraline
    B. Zolpidem
    C. Bupropion
    D. Paroxetine
    E. Lorazepam

End of set

155. A 68-year-old male with a long-standing history of bipolar disorder was recently discharged from the hospital. Tonight he is brought to the ED with gait problems, shoulder shaking, elbow rigidity, and tremor. Which of the following combinations of medications is most likely producing these symptoms?

    A. Fluphenazine and lithium
    B. Risperidone and lithium
    C. Risperidone and carbamazepine
    D. Risperidone and valproate
    E. Fluphenazine and benztropine

156. A 26-year-old graduate student presents to the university hospital ED complaining of insomnia for the past 2 weeks. She is quite distraught because finals are approaching and her poor sleep is making it hard to concentrate. After performing a careful history and examination, you are unable to identify any other problems, so you proceed to instruct her about good sleep hygiene. Which of the following tactics is consistent with that approach?

    A. Sleeping-in on the weekends
    B. Frequent naps
    C. Wind-down time between work and sleep
    D. Exercise just before bedtime
    E. Later dinner meals

The next three questions (items 157, 158, and 159) correspond to the following vignette.

A 20-year-old college sophomore is brought to the ED by her two roommates. She is tachycardic, hypertensive, and sweating, and she has dilated pupils. Her roommates inform the triage nurse that they were all at a rave dance club several hours before the patient became agitated and incoherent.

157. What is this patient's most likely diagnosis?

    A. Acute alcohol intoxication
    B. Acute alcohol withdrawal
    C. Ecstasy intoxication
    D. Marijuana inhalation
    E. LSD ingestion

158. What is the correct chemical name for the substance that this patient has taken?

    A. Ketanserin
    B. Olanzapine
    C. 3,4-Methylene dioxymethamphetamine
    D. D-lysergic acid
    E. Citalopram

159. Which of the following is an expected acute effect from intoxication with the substance that this patient has taken?

A. A sense of distance or aloofness toward others
B. Muscle relaxation
C. Increased appetite
D. Sleepiness
E. Decreased libido

End of set

---

160. A 26-year-old separated mother of two infant children has been brought to the emergency center by her older sister. The patient has bruises about her eyes, shoulders, and forearms. She is weeping profusely. In regard to the negative family consequences of substance abuse, which of the following statements is correct?

A. Serious neglect is present in few families with substance abuse.
B. Few male child abusers are substance abusers.
C. Most female child abusers are substance abusers.
D. Nearly half of the women treated for domestic violence drink alcohol heavily.
E. Few male domestic violence assailants drink heavily.

> **The next three questions (items 161, 162, and 163) correspond to the following vignette.**

A 33-year-old man embarking on a cross-country trip was hospitalized at a rural facility for religious grandiosity and extreme verbosity. He is transferred to the university hospital emergency center for further mental status changes, muscular rigidity, elevated temperature, and irregular heartbeats.

161. What is this patient's most likely diagnosis?

A. Manic delirium
B. Akathisia
C. Neuroleptic malignant syndrome
D. Pseudo-parkinsonism
E. Oculogyric crisis

162. Which of the following options is indicated in the management of this patient?

A. Dantrolene
B. Broad-spectrum antibiotics
C. Risperidone
D. Thioridazine
E. Fluid restriction

163. What of the following statements is true regarding this patient's diagnosis?

A. It is an uncommon but potentially fatal condition.
B. It is a common and potentially fatal condition.

C. It is a common and relatively benign condition.

D. It is an uncommon and relatively benign condition.

E. It is seen more frequently with atypical antipsychotic medications than with typical antipsychotic medications.

End of set

---

164. A 29-year-old Hispanic homemaker is persuaded to go to the emergency room by a girlfriend who is concerned that she has not left her home in the past 3 weeks. The patient admits that she typically avoids crowded places because she has a fear that she will accidentally urinate in public. This has never happened, but her anxiety about the possibility of this scenario has gotten so severe that she has had to rely on friends to do all of her errands, including grocery shopping. The patient has no history of urinary incontinence, nor any condition that would make this a likely event. When she is at home, she realizes that the likelihood of this event ever happening is close to nil. She denies any episodes of rapid-onset, severe anxiety accompanied by chest pain, shortness of breath, or fears of losing control. What is her most likely diagnosis?

A. Social phobia

B. Agoraphobia without history of panic disorder

C. Panic disorder with agoraphobia

D. Generalized anxiety disorder

E. Delusional disorder

The next two questions (items 165 and 166) correspond to the following vignette.

An 8-year-old girl is brought to the ED by her parents. The parents are bewildered because their daughter has been mute for the past 3 days. The girl's physical exam is normal.

165. What is the most likely diagnosis in this patient?

A. Catatonia

B. Stroke

C. Infection

D. Drugs

E. Elective mutism

166. Which of the following is the best approach in the management of a pediatric patient with mutism?

A. Prolonged interviewing

B. Elaborate mental status examination

C. Empathetic concern

D. Persistent and close-at-hand observation

E. Sedative-hypnotic medication

End of set

167. A 19-year-old college student returns to the emergency room 10 days after being sexually assaulted. Since the assault, she has had recurrent thoughts about the event. She finds it distressing to be in physical proximity to male strangers, even on a crowded street in broad daylight. She has experienced feelings of numbness and "being outside" her body. The patient makes an effort to avoid television shows involving crime and violence. She finds it difficult to sleep at night. Family and friends have remarked to her that she is much more irritable and "jumpy." Because of these symptoms, she has been unable to attend classes and avoids meeting friends at night. This individual meets the criteria for which of the following?

    A. Post-traumatic stress disorder
    B. Acute stress disorder
    C. Adjustment disorder with a mixture of depressed and anxious features
    D. Major depressive disorder
    E. Anxiety disorder not-otherwise-specified

The next two questions (items 168 and 169) correspond to the following vignette.

A 23-year-old woman is brought to the ED by her boyfriend. She is hyperreflexic, hallucinating, and practically insensitive to pain. Her boyfriend admits that both smoked a joint laced with phencyclidine (PCP) only hours before.

168. The proper management of PCP intoxication should include which of the following steps?

    A. Enhanced sensory stimulation
    B. Risperidone
    C. Fluoxetine
    D. Alkalinize urine
    E. Outpatient care

169. Which of the following is a common street name for PCP?

    A. Black beauties
    B. Angel dust
    C. Crack
    D. Horse
    E. Mother's little helpers

End of set

---

170. A man brings his wife to the emergency room complaining that she is "out of control." Her behavior changed when she stayed up several nights in a row trying to meet a deadline for her editor. Her sleep has been poor for the past 10 days. The patient is extremely talkative and jumps from topic to topic. She states loudly her plan to author the "greatest novel ever written" and sell it to the largest publishing houses. She has completely disrobed and is attempting to seduce her male nurse. She is very restless and shows extreme affective instability, with laughter often dissolving into crying. In the past year, her husband recalls two episodes lasting approximately 3 to 4 weeks at a time when the patient complained of overwhelming sadness and hopelessness. She

seemed uninterested in everything and lost weight due to her poor appetite. During these episodes, she was unable to function at work or at home. In between these depressive episodes there was a period that lasted about 3 or 4 days when the patient talked faster than usual, finished several chapters of her book, and slept for only a few hours at night. In the emergency room, a urine drug screen is negative. Physical exam and routine laboratory results, including TSH level, are normal. The patient has no history of medical problems and is not on any medications. Which of the following statements is true regarding this patient?

A. For a diagnosis of bipolar disorder, type I, to be made, an individual must have at least one manic episode lasting longer than 1 week and one depressive episode lasting at least 2 weeks.
B. Major depressive disorder would have a higher rate of transmission than would bipolar disorder if this couple requested counseling regarding the likelihood of their children having psychiatric illness.
C. This patient meets the criteria for bipolar disorder, type I, with rapid cycling.
D. Prognosis for bipolar disorder is usually better than in major depressive disorder, as patients tend to "burn out" as they age.
E. If this patient had significant hallucinations and delusions, she may have met the criteria for an official diagnosis of schizophrenia and bipolar disorder.

> **The next three questions (items 171, 172, and 173) correspond to the following vignette.**

A 28-year-old part-time carpet cleaner is brought to the ED by the police. He had been picked up outside a nearby convenience market where he was screaming obscenities at customers as they entered the store. On exam he is disheveled, unkempt, agitated, and wild-eyed.

171. Which of the following would constitute an improper reason for using restraints on this patient?

A. Prevention of imminent harm
B. For the convenience of staff
C. Decreasing stimulation
D. Prevention of disruption to the treatment setting
E. As a contingency in behavioral therapy

172. The best practice of subduing a patient by restraints includes which of the following?

A. Including only staff unfamiliar to the patient
B. A three-member restraining team
C. Debriefing
D. Limiting staff involvement to unit personnel
E. Oral medication

173. The means of restraining a pre-adolescent child typically includes which of the following?

A. A five-point restraining technique
B. Negotiation
C. Employing a holding technique
D. Surreptitiously placing medication in the patient's food beforehand
E. Asking involvement from the patient's peers

End of set

174. A 51-year-old retired postal worker is brought to the emergency room by a close friend for complaints of gross blood in the urine. He is diagnosed by the internist as having hypertrophy of the prostate, and follow-up is set up with a urologist. A psychiatric consultation is requested because the friend who accompanied the patient is worried about the patient's belief that the CIA is spying on him. The patient believes that his house is bugged and that the CIA has started to monitor his movements in his home by flying helicopters over his property at night. He denies having auditory or visual hallucinations, and his friend denies that the patient has shown any bizarre behavior. You diagnose him with delusional disorder. Which of the following statements is true regarding this patient's diagnosis?

A. For this diagnosis to be made, symptoms must be present for at least 1 month.
B. In delusional disorder, the delusional thinking is pervasive, affecting many aspects of the patient's life.
C. The subtype of delusional disorder in this man is best described as grandiose.
D. Even in delusional disorder with a significant depressive component, sole treatment with an antipsychotic for the major symptom of delusional thinking results in a better outcome than a more complicated regimen combining an antipsychotic with an antidepressant.
E. This disorder is mainly distinguishable from schizophrenia, paranoid type, by the time course of the symptoms.

175. A man is brought into the emergency room by police for treatment of various cuts and abrasions after he was assaulted by a neighbor for spying on the neighbor's wife as she undressed. The patient has had two previous brief incarcerations for similar infractions in the past 12 months. Which of the following statements is true regarding this patient's diagnosis of paraphilia?

A. One paraphilia is mutually exclusive of another paraphilia, making it inadvisable to ask about other possible behaviors.
B. Affected individuals typically are comfortable with self-disclosure of details regarding their behavior.
C. In paraphiliacs whose behavior harms others, cognitive therapy may play a role in treatment.
D. Paraphiliac fantasies are equivalent to paraphiliac disorders.
E. This patient exhibits a type of paraphilia known as frotteurism.

The next four questions (items 176–179) correspond to the following vignette.

A 26-year-old obese, part-time student with a long-standing history of paranoia is brought to the ED by his sister. She is concerned that her brother will act on his threats to harm their neighbor.

176. Which of the following court cases refers to the duty to warn?

A. *Rennie vs. Klein*
B. *Stone vs. Proctor*
C. *Blanchard vs. Levine*
D. *Tarasoff vs. Regents of University of California*
E. *Clifford vs. United States*

177. Regarding violent patients, which of the following statements is most correct?

A. Standards for assessment of risk factors do not exist.
B. Standards of care for the prediction of violent behavior do exist.
C. The clinician should assess the risk of violence frequently.
D. A risk-benefit assessment should be conducted after discharge.
E. The potential for violence is independent of the patient's mental state at any given time.

178. The "four D's" of malpractice include which one of the following?

A. Data
B. Deviation
C. Debenture
D. Drugs
E. Decree

179. Which of the more common allegations of psychiatric malpractice is claimed most frequently?

A. Undue familiarity
B. Incorrect treatment
C. Suicide
D. Incorrect diagnosis
E. Medication error

End of set

The next three questions (items 180, 181, and 182) correspond to the following vignette.

A 46-year-old homeless man was brought to the ED by paramedics. He was found lying face down and mumbling to himself at a nearby city park. As he is being placed on a gurney, one of the nurses relates, "I know this patient ... his name is Bill   last time he was here he went into DTs ..."

180. Which of the following characterizations of delirium tremens (DTs) is correct?

   A. Occurs in the majority of chronic alcoholics
   B. Usually begins 24 to 36 hours after the last drink
   C. Usually occurs in those who have been drinking heavily for 1 to 3 years
   D. May last 1 to 5 days
   E. If untreated, mortality is the rule

181. Which of the following diets is the best option in the treatment of this patient with impending DTs?

   A. Low-fat diet
   B. Low-calorie diet
   C. Salt-restricted diet
   D. High-calorie, high-carbohydrate diet
   E. High-protein, low-calorie diet

182. A complication of alcohol withdrawal is Wernicke-Korsakoff syndrome. Which of the following supplements is indicated to help prevent the syndrome from developing in this patient?

   A. Folate
   B. Multivitamins
   C. Vitamin B_{12}
   D. Magnesium
   E. Thiamine

End of set

The next two questions (items 183 and 184) correspond to the following vignette.

A 32-year-old former professional boxer is brought to the ED by paramedics. He was found obtunded in the alley next to a nearby convenience store. On examination, he has pinpoint pupils, bradycardia, depressed respiration, and hypothermia.

183. What is this patient's most likely diagnosis?

   A. Cocaine intoxication
   B. Alcohol intoxication
   C. Phencyclidine intoxication
   D. Benzodiazepine intoxication
   E. Opioid intoxication

184. Which pharmacologic intervention is indicated for the treatment of this patient's intoxication?

   A. Diazepam
   B. Flurazepam
   C. Naloxone

D. Haloperidol

E. Thiamine

End of set

---

185. A 32-year-old single woman comes into the emergency room complaining of fever that has persisted despite multiple trials of oral antibiotics. Her medical record reveals that she has an extensive history of hospitalizations and procedures. One of the residents who treated the patient during the past hospital stay confides that there has been previous suspicion that the woman is inducing these fevers by covert means for the sole purpose of obtaining medical attention. Which of the following statements is true regarding this patient's suspected diagnosis of factitious disorder?

A. Munchausen's syndrome is a less severe form of factitious disorder.

B. The patient benefits from or has external incentives for the production of signs or symptoms.

C. The symptoms in factitious disorder are unconsciously produced.

D. Patients with this diagnosis often have a background in a medically related field, and are typically educated, intelligent young women of a higher socioeconomic class.

E. Coexisting medical disease is, by definition, not a possibility with this diagnosis.

186. A 19-year-old soldier is triaged from the field for emergency treatment. He cannot remember the events of a skirmish in which most members of his squad were killed. Which of the following statements is true regarding this patient's diagnosis of dissociative amnesia?

A. It is more common in males than in females.

B. Its incidence is thought to increase during disasters.

C. This disorder is consciously motivated.

D. Substance abuse is rarely the cause of amnestic episodes.

E. Psychotropic medications are frequently useful in these episodes.

The next two questions (items 187 and 188) correspond to the following vignette.

A 32-year-old woman comes into the emergency room accompanied by her husband. She has recurrent thoughts and images of drowning her 3-week-old baby in the bathtub. The patient denies having auditory hallucinations commanding her to take this step, and is very distressed by these thoughts. Because of these thoughts and images, she excessively checks on her baby "to make sure he is safe." She denies having poor energy, tearfulness, irritability, periods of sadness, or mood lability. Physical examination reveals a healthy-appearing female who is clean and well groomed. The remainder of the exam and routine labs are unremarkable.

187. What is this patient's most likely diagnosis?

A. Postpartum blues

B. Postpartum depression

C. Puerperal psychosis

D. Adjustment disorder

E. Obsessive-compulsive disorder

188. Which of the following medications would be considered first-line treatment of the patient in the preceding clinical scenario?

    A. Sertraline
    B. Risperidone
    C. Haloperidol
    D. Lithium carbonate
    E. Valproic acid

End of set

189. A 19-year-old, HIV-positive waitress is brought to the emergency center by paramedics after she abruptly "passed out" at work. This is the fourth such episode in less than 3 months. Which of the following signs and symptoms is more likely in seizures than pseudo-seizures and will help confirm your diagnosis?

    A. Aura
    B. Secondary gain
    C. Affected by suggestion
    D. Asynchronous body movements
    E. Normal EEG

190. A 29-year-old man presents to the emergency center complaining of muscle aches, nausea, and vomiting. Physical exam reveals a fever of 101.4°F, diaphoresis, dilated pupils, and rhinorrhea. Which of the following abused substances is most likely responsible for this presentation?

    A. Alcohol
    B. Cocaine
    C. Amphetamines
    D. Heroin
    E. Phencyclidine (PCP)

The next two questions (items 191 and 192) correspond to the following vignette.

A 25-year-old homemaker accompanied by her husband is seen in the emergency room complaining of sudden loss of vision. Earlier that day she witnessed her son being hit by a car outside her home. During her neurological exam, she blinks when presented with visual threat. The remainder of her physical and neurological exam is normal. The patient's son sustained only minor fractures. Surprisingly, the patient denies any current anxiety and appears to be quite unconcerned by her loss of vision.

191. What is her most likely diagnosis?

    A. Post-traumatic stress disorder
    B. Conversion disorder
    C. Acute stress disorder
    D. Somatization disorder
    E. Histrionic personality disorder

192. Which of the following statements is true regarding treatment of this patient's disorder?

A. Studies have shown that confronting the patient results in the most rapid resolution of symptoms.
B. The presence of histrionic personality disorder, "la belle indifference," and secondary gain are sufficient to support a diagnosis of this disorder.
C. Estimates for prevalence of this disorder's symptoms are that it is very rare for patients admitted to a general medical setting.
D. Approximately one in five patients initially diagnosed with this disorder is later diagnosed with somatization disorder.
E. The deficit or symptom in this disorder is intentionally produced, as it is in malingering and factitious disorder.

End of set

193. A 33-year-old schoolteacher is brought to the emergency center after taking an overdose of her psychiatric medications. She is very irritable, complaining of diarrhea and on examination demonstrating myoclonus, elevated blood pressure, tachycardia, hyperpyrexia, and diaphoresis. Which of the following medications did she most likely take an overdose of?

A. Bupropion
B. Fluoxetine
C. Clozapine
D. Alprazolam
E. Diazepam

> **The next two questions (items 194 and 195) correspond to the following vignette.**

A 16-year-old girl is accompanied to the emergency center by her mother and stepfather. She is acting oddly and responding as if someone not visible to you is in the examination room. She is also grabbing her abdomen as if she is in pain. On physical exam, you are struck by her physical immaturity and a tremor. Screening labs are normal except for an anemia.

194. Which of the following metabolic diseases is the likely diagnosis?

A. Hypothyroidism
B. Wilson's disease
C. Hyperthyroidism
D. Hyperparathyroidism
E. Hypoparathyroidism

195. Which element is associated with the disease described in this vignette?

  A. Calcium
  B. Phosphorus
  C. Copper
  D. Iron
  E. Sodium

End of set

196. A 53-year-old attorney with a history of episodic alcohol abuse presents to the emergency center with ataxia and confusion. His clothes smell of urine. He vomits and then has a tonic-clonic seizure and becomes unresponsive. His wife is present and thinks he may have overdosed on his medication. Which medication would be most likely to cause his symptoms?

  A. Gabapentin
  B. Valproic acid
  C. Fluphenazine
  D. Lithium carbonate
  E. Clonazepam

197. A 68-year-old widower with severe rheumatoid arthritis and hypertension has been transported by the paramedics to the emergency center. His neighbors found him sitting on his front porch, mumbling and disoriented. Which of the following symptoms, if exhibited, would be considered the hallmark for a diagnosis of delirium?

  A. Fluctuating mental status
  B. Visual hallucinations
  C. Illusions
  D. Disorientation
  E. Affective symptoms

The next two questions (items 198 and 199) correspond to the following vignette.

A 22-year-old Asian student is brought to the university hospital emergency center by her parents. The patient is very distressed, believing both her parents are imposters and involved in a complicated scheme to control the young woman's life. The remainder of the mental status examination is normal, and a urine drug screen is negative.

198. What is this patient's most likely diagnosis?

  A. Folie á deux
  B. Capgras' syndrome
  C. Schizophrenia, paranoid type
  D. Depersonalization disorder
  E. Dissociative identity disorder (DID)

199. The medical student accompanying you during the examination asks you to tell her more about DID. Which of the following characterizations is correct regarding DID?

A. The number of reported cases has been decreasing
B. Often presents after age 40
C. Is frequently associated with substance abuse
D. Cannot be helped with hypnosis
E. Is frequently helped by medications

End of set

200. A 53-year-old airport security guard is brought to the emergency center by her spouse. You are asked to provide psychiatric consultation because she is irritable, paranoid, and depressed. During your examination of the patient, you are struck by her dry skin, Parkinsonian-like faces, and cogwheel rigidity of her arms. Which of the following endocrine disorders should be included in your differential diagnosis?

A. Addison's disease
B. Cushing's syndrome
C. Hyperparathyroidism
D. Hypoparathyroidism
E. Hyperthyroidism

Answers and Explanations

151. D	168. B	185. D
152. B	169. B	186. B
153. A	170. C	187. E
154. E	171. B	188. A
155. A	172. C	189. A
156. C	173. C	190. D
157. C	174. A	191. B
158. C	175. C	192. D
159. C	176. D	193. B
160. D	177. C	194. B
161. C	178. B	195. C
162. A	179. B	196. D
163. A	180. D	197. A
164. B	181. D	198. B
165. E	182. E	199. C
166. C	183. E	200. D
167. B	184. C	

151. **D.** Chest pain, diaphoresis, hot flashes, shortness of breath, and fear of dying can all be symptoms of panic disorder. Other symptoms of panic may include palpitations, tremulousness, choking, nausea, dizziness, numbness or tingling, chills, feelings of unreality and depersonalization, and fear of going crazy. The rapid onset and short duration are also consistent with a panic attack.

A. Somatic delusions typically involve concern about parasites, an altered self-image, or fears of giving off a foul body odor. These symptoms must be present consistently for 1 month to make a diagnosis.

B. PTSD is incorrect. There is no evidence that the patient's symptoms are a result of trauma.

C. Although anxiety is also a central feature in OCD, no evidence indicates that the patient had been experiencing recurrent or persistent obsessional thoughts or compulsive behaviors.

E. The patient's symptoms follow a time frame more consistent with a panic disorder in that they are acute, relatively brief, and episodic, unlike the persistent, long-term symptoms of GAD.

152. **B.** Agoraphobia, or fear of open spaces, is most closely associated with panic disorder. The other four phobias can be found in persons with panic disorder but are not as prevalent.

A. Apiphobia is the fear of bees.

C. Claustrophobia is the fear of enclosed spaces.

D. Gynophobia is the fear of women.

E. Hydrophobia is the fear of water.

153. **A.** Thyroid function testing is routinely used to rule out hyperthyroidism. Patients with hyperthyroidism can present with symptoms similar to panic disorder.

B. Fasting glucose is not a routine test in the work-up of panic disorder, although hypoglycemia may cause similar symptoms.

C. Plasma cortisol is not a routine test in the work-up of panic disorder.

D. Testing of testosterone levels is not indicated in the work-up of panic disorder.

E. Arterial blood gases are not routinely measured in the evaluation of panic disorder. If the patient's symptoms persisted or there was evidence of a cardiac or pulmonary condition, such tests could be pursued.

154. **E.** Lorazepam is a fast-acting benzodiazepine that is most appropriate for patients for acute management of panic symptoms.

A. Sertraline, a selective serotonin reuptake inhibitor (SSRI), is useful in the long-term management of panic disorder but will have no immediate beneficial effects for patients.

B. Zolpidem, a non-benzodiazepine hypnotic, is used for the short-term management of insomnia.

C. Bupropion, a selective dopamine reuptake inhibitor (SDRI), is not typically used for first-line treatment of panic disorder.

D. Paroxetine, an SSRI, is useful in the long-term management of panic disorder but will have no immediate beneficial effects for patients.

155. **A.** Typical, or first-generation, antipsychotics such as fluphenazine in combination with lithium frequently cause extrapyramidal symptoms (EPS). Their synergistic therapeutic effect likely also causes this side effect, which is more common in elderly patients.

B. The atypical antipsychotic risperidone combined with lithium is generally well tolerated.

C. Risperidone plus carbamazepine is often well tolerated, although discontinuation of the carbamazepine may elevate the risperidone level and produce EPS.

D. Risperidone combined with valproate is well tolerated.

E. Presumably, the anticholinergic agent benztropine combined with fluphenazine would prevent EPS.

156. **C.** Allowing some wind-down time is important before going to bed.

A. Sleep hygiene includes maintaining a consistent bedtime and wake-up schedule, even on weekends.

B. Good sleep hygiene includes avoiding naps or at least keeping them short.

D. Exercise, but not within 3 hours of going to bed, is considered important to promote good sleep.

E. Good sleep hygiene includes avoiding heavy eating as well as consumption of tobacco, alcohol, and caffeine near bedtime.

157. **C.** Ecstasy is an increasingly popular "club drug" that is often used at all-night dance parties and clubs. The patient's clinical presentation resembles amphetamine toxicity.

A. Alcohol intoxication would not result in tachycardia and dilated pupils but more likely vomiting and a strong odor of alcohol.

B. Alcohol withdrawal typically takes many hours after the last drink in a chronically dependent person and is unlikely to cause dilated pupils.

D. Marijuana ingestion is unlikely to result in such a severe physiologic response.

E. LSD, another "club drug," tends not to result in such severe physiologic changes.

158. **C.** 3,4-Methylene dioxymethamphetamine (MDMA) is the chemical name for the club drug Ecstasy. As its name implies, Ecstasy is an amphetamine derivative.

A. Ketanserin is a serotonin antagonist, which, if given before exposure to Ecstasy, can attenuate the response.

B. Olanzapine is an atypical antipsychotic with serotonin- and dopamine-blocking properties.

D. D-Lysergic acid is a hallucinogen, better known as LSD.

E. Citalopram is a serotonergic antidepressant that may attenuate some of the psychological effects of Ecstasy.

159. **C.** During acute intoxication from Ecstasy, an increased appetite is common but anorexia may follow.

A. Reported positive effects from Ecstasy include decreased defensiveness and a decreased sense of alienation rather than increased distance or aloofness.

B. Trismus, or jaw clenching, as well as teeth grinding occur with Ecstasy use.

D. Sleepiness and decreased motivation and fatigue are not experienced during acute intoxication with Ecstasy but rather are after-effects experienced the next day or later.

E. Sexual arousal and increased libido are sought-after positive effects from Ecstasy.

160. **D.** Approximately 50% of women treated for domestic violence were drinking heavily.

A. Serious neglect is present in more than 40% of drug-abusing families.

B. More than 40% of male child abusers are substance abusers.

C. Approximately 30% of female child abusers are substance abusers.

E. Nearly 90% of male domestic violence assailants were drinking heavily.

161. **C.** Neuroleptic malignant syndrome (NMS) is the likely diagnosis. The clinical history suggests an acute manic episode, necessitating hospitalization in the rural setting and likely exposure to antipsychotic medications as an acute intervention.

A. It is quite possible that the mania remains but the physical abnormalities are consistent with NMS.

B. Akathisia is a subjective sense of jitteriness experienced with antipsychotic medications.

D. Pseudo-parkinsonism or EPS would not have the constellation of findings, including rigidity, hyperthermia, and arrhythmia, associated with NMS.

E. Oculogyric crisis is a specific acute dystonia associated with antipsychotic medications.

162. **A.** Dantrolene, a skeletal muscle relaxant, can lessen the rigidity and hyperthermia of NMS.

B. An underlying or concurrent infection is not uncommon in the pathogenesis of NMS, but a specific organism should be identified first as fever is part of the syndrome as well.

C. Risperidone and all other antipsychotics are contraindicated in the management of NMS.

D. Thioridazine, an antipsychotic, is contraindicated in the management of NMS.

E. The hyperthermia, elevated CPK associated with muscular rigidity, and other symptoms all warrant aggressive fluid management.

163. | **A.** NMS is an uncommon but potentially fatal illness. Approximately 0.2% of patients exposed to typical antipsychotics develop NMS of varying severity. Nearly 40% of patients with NMS develop significant physical complications, and as many as 20% die.

B, C, D. See the explanation for A.

E. NMS was much more common with the typical antipsychotic medications such as the phenothiazines and haloperidol.

164. | **B.** The diagnosis is agoraphobia without history of panic disorder. This patient has markedly restricted her normal activities due to a fear that she will develop urinary incontinence in public. Agoraphobia is the fear of being in situations from which escape might be difficult if the person develops an embarrassing or incapacitating symptom. More rarely, there is no history of panic disorder, and the fear relates to developing some specific symptoms such as urinary incontinence, vomiting, or cardiac distress.

A. Social phobia is a persistent fear of a situation in which a person is exposed to possible scrutiny by others. In this disorder, the individual is trying to accomplish a voluntary activity (e.g., speaking, writing, eating, urinating) and fears that this activity will be impaired by signs of anxiety (e.g., stuttering, being tremorous while writing, being too self-conscious to urinate). By contrast, in agoraphobia without a history of panic disorder, the individual is afraid of suddenly developing a symptom that is unrelated to the activity he or she is attempting to accomplish.

C. Usually agoraphobia is diagnosed as a qualifier of panic disorder, in which a person avoids certain situations that are associated with having panic symptoms. In this patient, there is no history of symptoms indicating the occurrence of unprovoked panic attacks.

D. This patient has a very specific anxiety, whereas generalized anxiety disorder is characterized by excessive worry about everyday things more than in the average person.

E. A delusion is a fixed, false belief. In contrast, when this individual is not in a public place she has the insight to acknowledge that her thinking is not logical. Insight is typically poor in a person with delusional disorder.

165. | **E.** In children, mutism is more often than not elective. In young adults, it may arise from a multitude of conditions including psychiatric conditions. In older patients, a top concern would be a neurologic condition.

A. Catatonia associated with schizophrenia and mood disorders can be manifested as mutism. Although not the most likely diagnoses in an 8-year-old, these possibilities would be included in the differential diagnosis.

B. A neurologic condition such as stroke would be unusual in a child, especially without other physical findings.

C. A CNS infection could cause mutism but other symptoms would be expected as well.

D. Sedating agents can cause mutism as well as a variety of abused drugs such as hallucinogens. This diagnosis would be less likely in a child.

166. C. Empathetic nursing staff who are with the patient for extensive periods may gain more information.

A. Frequent but brief contacts are more useful than a prolonged interview.

B. Simple, concrete questions are more likely to evoke responses.

D. Surreptitious observation may reveal a malingering aspect or other odd behavior.

E. Often there is an underlying psychosis, so antipsychotic medications are the preferred treatment.

167. B. Acute stress disorder lasts between 2 days and 4 weeks. This patient shows a reexperiencing symptom ("recurrent thoughts about the event"), avoidance symptoms (violent television shows and meeting friends at night), and hyperarousal symptoms (being jumpy and finding it difficult to sleep at night) with onset after a traumatic event.

A. A time period of at least 4 weeks is required for a diagnosis of PTSD, as well as at least one reexperiencing symptom, three avoidance symptoms, and two hyperarousal symptoms.

C. The time course of adjustment disorder involves symptoms that appear within 3 months of a significant event, but then resolve by 6 months after the event. In adjustment disorder, the event that caused the change in mood must be something that may be experienced by the average person during his or her lifetime, such as the loss of a job or the end of a relationship. A violent assault does not fit into this category.

D. Although this patient does have some depressive symptoms, the fact that a traumatic episode that could have led to severe bodily harm or even death precipitated the symptoms is more indicative of an acute stress disorder. Another clue that would eliminate a diagnosis of clinical depression is the time course of 10 days; the time course for major depression is at least 2 weeks.

E. Acute stress disorder is a type of anxiety disorder, but enough details are presented in the history to allow for a more accurate diagnosis of acute stress disorder.

168. B. Psychotic symptoms should be actively treated with an antipsychotic medication such as risperidone

A. Sensory stimulation should be minimized; attempts to reassure the patient may aggravate the situation.

C. An antidepressant such as fluoxetine is not indicated in the treatment of PCP intoxication.

D. The urine should be acidified to increase excretion with ascorbic acid or ammonium chloride.

E. The patient should be monitored closely because large ingestions may result in seizures, coma, and death. Hospitalization is usually indicated.

---

169. **B.** Although relying on street jargon to correctly discern which drugs have been ingested is precarious, the nickname "angel dust" is commonly associated with PCP.

A. "Black beauties" typically refers to stimulants.

C. "Crack" refers to cocaine.

D. "Horse" refers to heroin.

E. "Mother's little helpers" commonly refers to sedative-hypnotics and benzodiazepines.

---

170. **C.** According to the husband's history, in the past year the patient has had a depressed episode, a hypomanic episode, another depressed episode, and now a full-blown manic episode. Thus the patient meets the requirement for four or more mood cycles in a 1-year period to warrant the qualifier "with rapid cycling." Rapid cycling usually involves one or more manic or hypomanic episodes, but is also diagnosed if all the episodes are depressed, manic, or hypomanic as long as they are separated by periods of remission (or switches to the opposite pole). This qualifier is of clinical relevance, as patients with rapid-cycling bipolar disorder have high rates of nonresponse to lithium. Outcomes may be more successful if the disorder is treated with anticonvulsants, such as carbamazepine or valproic acid.

A. This patient shows rapid speech, decreased need for sleep, grandiosity, hyperactivity, hypersexuality, and a suggestion of loose associations and flight of ideas. A single manic episode is sufficient for a diagnosis of bipolar disorder, type I.

B. Studies have shown that bipolar disorder has a higher rate of genetic transmission than both major depressive disorder and schizophrenia. In fact, the risk of bipolar disorder transmission is 60% for people with two parents with bipolar disorder, 20% for first-degree relatives of patients with bipolar disorder, and 1% for the general population.

D. Bipolar disorder tends to carry a worse prognosis than major depressive disorder, with episodes of depression or mania occurring closer in time as a person ages.

E. When patients or well-meaning family members give a confusing history of multiple diagnoses, including schizophrenia and bipolar disorder in the same individual, it indicates a lack of communication and education by the patient's treating professional. It may also result from different diagnoses being made by different individuals at different times in the person's life. Interestingly, although no ethnic differences have been found in the occurrence of bipolar disorder, in African

American and Hispanic patients of low socioeconomic class, bipolar disorders are often misdiagnosed as schizophrenia. A mixture of mood and psychotic symptoms should be explored in depth to differentiate among a possibility of diagnoses; some examples would be major depressive disorder, severe with psychotic features, or schizoaffective disorder, bipolar subtype. Until clarification can be made, it is best to assign a diagnosis of psychosis not-otherwise-specified or mood disorder not-otherwise-specified to avoid further confusion.

171. | **B.** Restraints are improperly used for the convenience of the staff or to punish a patient. The expectation is to provide care in the least restrictive environment.

A. Restraining for the prevention of imminent harm to the patient or staff is indicated if other means such as medication or verbal interventions are ineffective.

C. The agitated, labile patient may require restraints until he or she can be placed in a less stimulating environment than the ED.

D. Restraints are indicated to prevent substantial damage or disruption to the setting. The confined space of an ED may require such measures.

E. Restraining a patient may serve as a contingency to help eliminate disruptive or dangerous behavior.

172. | **C.** The team, ideally with input from an observer, should critique the intervention with debriefing. This is instructional for the staff as well as helps them work through antecedent distress on their part.

A. Including a staff member familiar with the patient may be more comforting to the patient.

B. A five-member team is more appropriate to restrain a patient—one person for each limb and a team leader who also manages the patient's head.

D. Back-up resources—perhaps hospital security—as a show of force can be helpful in encouraging the patient to comply with the intervention.

E. More often than not, once the patient is securely in restraints, providing injectable medication is necessary and should be quickly available to help diminish the inappropriate behavior, agitation, psychosis, or other troublesome symptoms. Oral medications may be offered once the patient becomes cooperative and is able to swallow safely.

173. | **C.** Pre-adolescent children are not generally restrained in the same manner as larger teenagers or adults. A firm hugging of the child from behind as the patient's arms are held securely to each side may suffice.

A. The five-member team approach is reserved for larger or markedly agitated younger patients.

B. Once the decision to restrain a patient is made, negotiation may merely lead to further escalation.

D. Medications should not be given to patients surreptitiously.

E. Patient peer involvement is contraindicated.

174. **A.** Delusional disorder, formerly termed "paranoia," is a type of psychotic disorder characterized by a nonbizarre, fixed delusional system of at least 1 month's duration. The delusion is nonbizarre, meaning that it involves a situation that can occur in real life, such as being followed, infected, loved at a distance, and so forth. Although the phenomenon that is purported to occur is not real or likely, it is nevertheless possible.

B. The delusional thinking is circumscribed, not affecting other aspects of the patient's life. Although these patients may appear odd, eccentric, or reclusive, they usually remain outside of hospital settings because they may experience little impairment. Contact with professionals may be more likely related to litigation or general medical problems, as these individuals actively oppose psychiatric treatment and often have poor insight into their illness.

C. The subtypes of delusional disorder are erotomanic, grandiose, jealous, persecutory, somatic, and mixed. A delusion of the grandiose type focuses on possessing inflated worth, power, knowledge, identity, or a special relationship to a deity or famous person. This patient's delusion is best described as persecutory, in which the central theme is that the individual (or someone to whom the individual is close) is being attacked, harassed, cheated, persecuted, or conspired against.

D. Studies indicate that treatment of both the psychotic and the mood symptoms results in an improved outcome. This would also be true in other disorders, such as major depressive disorder with psychotic features.

E. While the time course for delusional disorder (at least 4 weeks) does differ from schizophrenia (at least 6 months), these two conditions are also distinguishable in another way—in delusional disorder there is an absence of bizarre delusions, hallucinations, or disorganized speech and behavior.

175. **C.** Paraphiliacs may engage in a variety of distortions to assuage the guilt they feel about the behavior, such as blaming the victim ("he/she made me do it") or denying the effects on the victim ("I could tell he/she enjoyed it"). Challenging belief systems may involve treatment programs that utilize testimony written by the victim or videos presented from the victim's standpoint.

A. Paraphilias are characterized by the preferential use of unusual objects of sexual desire or engagement in unusual sexual activity over a period of at least 6 months, causing impairment in occupational or social functioning. Some types of paraphilias are fetishism, frotteurism, pedophilia, and exhibitionism. Multiple paraphilias may be present in the same individual. Thus, when one paraphilia is known, one should screen for other paraphilias.

B. A clinician should never rely solely on report of symptoms by the patient, particularly when the behavior may inflict harm on others. An attempt to obtain corroborative information is necessary in any case of paraphilia.

D. Unless they are recurrent or intense, paraphilic fantasies are not paraphilias but simply normal components of human sexuality.

E. This individual exhibits a disorder called voyeurism, in which a person obtains sexual pleasure from secretly watching people (often with binoculars) undressing or engaging in sexual activity. In contrast, frotteurism is diagnosed when a person has recurrent urges over a 6-month period to rub against or touch a nonconsenting individual, for the purpose of sexual excitation, and either is distressed by these urges or has acted on them.

176. **D.** *Tarasoff vs. Regents of University of California* and related cases resulted in a ruling in most jurisdictions that a physician has the duty to warn or protect potential victims.

A. *Rennie vs. Klein* dealt with a patient's right to refuse treatment.

B *Stone vs. Proctor* dealt with standards of care.

C. *Blanchard vs. Levine* dealt with failure to evaluate a patient before administrating medications.

E. *Clifford vs. United States* dealt with the expectation to monitor patients receiving psychotropic medications.

177. **C.** The clinician should assess the risk for violence frequently and during critical junctures for treatment (e.g., granting of passes, discharge).

A. Professional standards do exist for the assessment of risk factors.

B. There is no standard of care (care is not the same as assessment) for predicting violent behavior.

D. A risk-benefit assessment should be conducted and documented *before* discharge.

E. The potential for violence is dependent on the patient's mental state and concurrent situational factors.

178. **B.** The "four D's" of malpractice include duty, deviation, damage, and direct causation.

A, C, D, E. See the explanation for B.

179. **B.** Incorrect treatment is claimed most frequently, accounting for 33% of psychiatric malpractice cases.

A. Allegations of undue familiarity account for approximately 3% of psychiatric malpractice claims.

C. Suicide and attempted suicide claims account for 20% of psychiatric malpractice cases.

D. Incorrect diagnosis is claimed in 11% of psychiatric malpractice cases.

E. Medication error and drug reactions are claimed in 7% of psychiatric malpractice cases.

180. **D.** DTs may last 1 to 5 days.

A. DTs occur in fewer than 5% of chronic alcoholics.

B. DTs usually begin 48 to 96 hours after cessation or decrease in alcohol intake.

C. DTs usually occur in those who have been drinking heavily for 5 to 15 years.

E. Left untreated, DTs may have a mortality rate as high as 20%.

181. **D.** The patient with impending DTs should be placed on a high-calorie, high-carbohydrate diet.

A, B, C, E. These are not the best diets in the treatment of impending DTs.

182. **E.** Thiamine deficiency is thought to be the cause of Wernicke's encephalopathy.

A. Folate deficiency is common in chronic alcoholics, but is not the cause of Wernicke's encephalopathy.

B. Vitamin deficiencies in general are common in chronic alcoholics.

C. Vitamin B_{12} deficiency does not cause Wernicke's encephalopathy.

D. Magnesium is sometimes used to ward off seizures, but does not treat Wernicke's encephalopathy.

183. **E.** Opioids include opium, morphine, heroin, meperidine, methadone, pentazocine, and propoxyphene. The pinpoint pupils are unresponsive to light.

A. Cocaine and other stimulant intoxication results in restlessness, tachycardia, and dilated reactive pupils.

B. Alcohol intoxication typically causes tachycardia, not bradycardia.

C. Phencyclidine intoxication causes tachycardia and nystagmus.

D. Benzodiazepine intoxication does not alter pupillary response; rather, it resembles alcohol intoxication.

184. **C.** Naloxone 0.4 to 2.0 mg IV every 2 to 3 minutes until respirations are stable is the antidote for opioid intoxication.

A. Diazepam, as a benzodiazepine, may worsen the patient's respiratory status.

B. Flurazepam, a benzodiazepine, is primarily used to promote sleep.

D. Haloperidol, as an antipsychotic, is not indicated and may complicate this patient's physical status.

E. Thiamine is used in alcohol withdrawal states.

185. **D.** Having a background in a medically related field allows these individuals to feign symptoms that are initially plausible. Affected persons are typically educated, intelligent individuals.

A. Munchausen's syndrome is a severe form of factitious disorder in which the person tends to wander from hospital to hospital and to change health care practitioners frequently to escape detection of the feigned illness.

B. Unlike malingering patients, the patient with factitious disorder does not benefit from or have external incentives for the production of signs or symptoms. The main goal is to assume the sick role.

C. The symptoms in factitious disorder are consciously produced, but the motivations for the clinical presentation are unconscious and should be addressed in therapy in this manner.

E. True illness may very well be present in a person with factitious disorder, particularly given that these individuals are often the recipients of well-intentioned diagnostic procedures that may result in complications (for example, the formation of adhesions after exploratory surgery). A thorough physical exam and lab work-up should always be done, but reservation should be used when considering invasive diagnostic procedures.

186. B. The incidence of dissociative amnesia is believed to rise during disasters, and this condition may affect as many as 5% to 8% of combat soldiers during wartime.

A. Dissociative amnesia is most common in adolescent and young adult females; it is most rare in the elderly.

C. The psychoanalytic model describes dissociative amnesia as unconsciously motivated. A memory may be so traumatic or laden with conflict that conscious awareness of it would be accompanied by insupportable anxiety. Therefore, the mind activates defense mechanisms such as repression and dissociation to keep the memory from entering conscious awareness.

D. Alcohol and hallucinogen abuse (as well as withdrawal syndromes) must be ruled out when confronted with memory disturbance in an individual. The "alcoholic blackout" is the classic substance-induced amnesia.

E. Psychotropic medications are rarely useful in the treatment of dissociative amnesia. Therapy relies on two principles: (1) removing the patient from the threatening circumstances by hospitalization if needed, and (2) addressing the emotional distress through psychotherapy.

187. E. Obsessive-compulsive disorder (OCD) is a type of anxiety disorder. Patients experience recurrent intrusive, unwanted feelings, thoughts, and images (obsessions) that cause marked anxiety and are to some extent relieved by performing repetitive actions (compulsions). The postpartum period may represent a time of increased risk for the development of OCD.

A. Although this patient is postpartum with the onset of symptoms within 4 weeks after delivery, she does not meet the criteria for postpartum blues, in which women experience mild depressive symptoms during the first week after delivery. This patient denies depressive symptoms other than the distress caused by the recurrent ego dystonic thoughts. Symptoms indicative of "the blues" include dysphoria, mood lability, irritability, tearfulness, anxiety, and insomnia.

B. Postpartum depression is a diagnosis made when a patient meets the criteria for major depressive disorder, with onset of the depressive episode occurring within 4 weeks postpartum.

C. Puerperal psychosis is the most severe form of postpartum psychiatric illness. Puerperal psychosis is rare, affecting approximately 1 to 2 women per 1000 mothers postpartum. Psychotic symptoms and disorganized behavior are observable and cause significant dysfunction. The psychosis is often sudden, appearing within 2 to

4 weeks after delivery, and may include auditory hallucinations or delusions that the child is somehow defective. An affective psychosis is often present.

D. Although having a child is certainly a significant life stressor, the prominent obsessional thoughts make the diagnosis of OCD more appropriate in this case.

188. A. SSRIs are considered first-line agents for the treatment of OCD. Other options besides sertraline are fluoxetine, paroxetine, citalopram, escitalopram, and fluvoxamine. Clomipramine, a mixed-action agent with potent serotonergic effects, was the first medication found to have an effect on OCD. It is now considered second-line therapy, because the dose titration needed to achieve a therapeutic effect often results in intolerable drowsiness and weight gain.

B. Risperidone, an antipsychotic, should not routinely be used to treat OCD.

C. Haloperidol, an antipsychotic, is not indicated for OCD.

D. Lithium carbonate, a mood stabilizer, is primarily used to treat bipolar disorder but not OCD.

E. Valproic acid, an anticonvulsant with mood-stabilizing properties, is not routinely used for OCD.

189. A. Auras are common in organic seizures but not in pseudo-seizures. The pseudo-seizure patient has some conscious control over mimicking the signs and symptoms of a seizure.

B. Secondary gain should arouse suspicion for pseudo-seizures.

C. Suggestibility should arouse suspicion for pseudo-seizures.

D. Asynchronous body movements should arouse suspicion for pseudo-seizures.

E. A normal EEG should arouse suspicion for pseudo-seizures.

190. D. Withdrawal from opioids such as heroin will present clinically with nausea, muscle aches, rhinorrhea, pupillary dilation, sweating, fever, and diarrhea. Treatment options include symptomatic stabilization with tapering doses of methadone.

A. Patients with alcohol withdrawal usually present with agitation, tremors, and elevated vital signs. Alcohol withdrawal would not explain this patient's dilated pupils or rhinorrhea.

B, C. Stimulants such as cocaine or amphetamines would cause agitation and elevated vital signs during intoxication, but usually cause the patient to develop somnolence and dysphoria upon withdrawal. Neither stimulant would explain all of this patient's symptoms. This patient's clinical presentation is more consistent with opioid withdrawal than with either stimulant intoxication or withdrawal.

E. Patients suffering from PCP intoxication typically are agitated, are combative, may demonstrate psychotic symptoms, and have a decreased sensitivity to pain. These symptoms are not consistent with this patient's clinical presentation.

191. **B.** This individual suffers from conversion disorder, in which there is an abrupt, dramatic loss of motor or sensory function suggestive of a neurological or medical condition. However, psychological factors are deemed the cause of the illness, as the loss of function is typically preceded by a particular stressor and may have symbolic significance.

A. To meet criteria A in DSM-IV for PTSD, an individual must have been exposed to a traumatic event. Further diagnostic criteria require a "1-3-2" symptom cluster (referring to criteria B, C, and D in DSM-IV): one reexperiencing symptom, three avoidance symptoms, and two hyperarousal symptoms. PTSD is categorized as an anxiety disorder. This patient denies any anxiety symptoms that would fit criteria B, C, or D for PTSD and, in fact, displays "la belle indifference" that is typical of conversion disorder. The time course for diagnosis of PTSD is greater than 4 weeks.

C. In acute stress disorder, the criteria are essentially the same as those in PTSD except that the time course lasts from 2 days to 4 weeks. Another contrast between acute stress disorder and PTSD is that only a "1-1-1" symptom cluster is required: at least one reexperiencing symptom, one avoidance symptom, and one hyperarousal symptom.

D. Diagnosis of somatization disorder requires a "4-2-1-1" symptom cluster: four gastrointestinal symptoms, two non-gastrointestinal pain symptoms, one pseudo-sexual symptom, and one pseudo-neurological symptom.

E. This patient is not exhibiting any of the symptoms of histrionic personality disorder.

192. **D.** When a symptom occurs in isolation, it is appropriate to make the diagnosis of conversion disorder. However, conversion symptoms may also occur as a component of other major syndromes, including somatization disorder, schizophrenia, depression, and even general medical or neurological disease.

A. Confrontation is not considered beneficial. Rather, suggestion of cure typically results in eventual resolution of the symptom or deficit.

B. Several traditional clinical features previously associated with conversion, such as secondary gain, histrionic personality, and "la belle indifference," have been shown to have little diagnostic significance. These are considered "soft signs" assisting in a possible diagnosis but having no concrete diagnostic validity. The diagnosis of conversion must ultimately rest on positive clinical findings clearly demonstrating that the etiology of the symptom is not physical disease.

C. Conversion symptoms are actually relatively common in medical practice, especially among patients admitted to a general medical setting.

E. The deficit or symptom in conversion disorder is not intentionally produced or feigned, in contrast to malingering and factitious disorder.

193. **B.** Fluoxetine is a serotonergic antidepressant. This patient's signs and symptoms of irritability; diarrhea; elevated blood pressure, pulse, and temperature; and diaphoresis are typical of a serotonin syndrome.

A. An overdose with the dopaminergic antidepressant bupropion would cause nausea, vomiting, dry mouth, and possibly seizures.

C. An overdose of the antipsychotic clozaril would likely cause postural hypotension, sedation, hypersalivation, constipation, and possibly seizures.

D. An overdose of the benzodiazepine alprazolam would likely cause drowsiness, ataxia, hypotension, bradycardia, and respiratory depression.

E. An overdose of the benzodiazepine diazepam would have much the same effects as described in the explanation for D.

194. **B.** Wilson's disease, or hepatolenticular degeneration, can present with a variety of psychiatric symptoms, including psychosis, as well as the physical sequelae associated with impaired hepatic function.

A. Hypothyroidism can also occur in adolescence. The psychiatric symptoms can be those seen in other endocrine or metabolic diseases but the physical findings are quite different, including dry, cold skin and bradycardia.

C. Hyperthyroidism usually occurs later in life (e.g., the fourth or fifth decade) and has different physical findings such as tachycardia; warm, moist skin; and tremor.

D. Hyperparathyroidism typically occurs in the 50- to 60-year-old age group and has physical symptoms expected with hypercalcemia.

E. Hypoparathyroidism can occur at any age. It has similar psychiatric symptoms but different physical findings than those associated with hypocalcemia.

195. **C.** Copper excess is associated with Wilson's disease.

A. Calcium is associated with parathyroid disease.

B. Phosphorus is also associated with parathyroid disease.

D. Iron deficiency is associated with anemia.

E. Sodium is associated with inappropriate antidiuretic syndrome as well as many other conditions.

196. **D.** The hallmarks of lithium toxicity include ataxia, tremor, confusion, vomiting, and urinary incontinence. Overdose with lithium carbonate can also lead to coma and seizures.

A. Gabapentin, an anticonvulsant, may cause confusion and ataxia in overdose, but would not cause urinary incontinence or seizures.

B. Valproic acid is an anticonvulsant with mood-stabilizing properties; the symptoms experienced with its toxicity or overdose are similar to those observed with gabapentin overdose.

C. Fluphenazine, a phenothiazine antipsychotic, may cause sedation and convulsions in overdose, but its anticholinergic effects would cause urinary retention.

E. Benzodiazepines, such as clonazepam, have anticonvulsant properties, so overdose would not cause seizures.

197. **A.** Fluctuating mental status is the hallmark of delirium.

B. Visual hallucinations can occur in every psychotic syndrome but suggest an organic etiology and are a common form of hallucinations in delirium.

C. Illusions are associated with the sensory misperception experienced in delirium but are not specific to that syndrome.

D. Disorientation is frequently seen in patients with delirium as well as in dementia, head injury, mental retardation, and other conditions.

E. Affective symptoms such as depression, irritability, and mania are seen in delirium but are not very specific to the condition.

198. **B.** Capgras' syndrome is a nonspecific delusion implying that the patient believes family members have been replaced by imposters. It can exist independent of more extensive psychiatric illness or can be a component of schizophrenia, dementia, and other syndromes with psychotic symptoms.

A. Folie á deux is a delusion shared between two people.

C. Schizophrenia is too broad a diagnosis for this patient because the patient lacks other specific symptoms typical of that illness.

D. Depersonalization is the experience of detachment from oneself; a true disorder implies persistent symptoms.

E. DID is also known as multiple personality disorder.

199. **C.** DID is frequently associated with substance abuse.

A. There has been a rise in reported cases of DID, perhaps related to mental health professionals' increased awareness of the disorder.

B. DID typically emerges between adolescence and the twenties; it can occur in childhood but rarely presents as a new disorder after age 40.

D. Hypnosis can be helpful in facilitating access to associated personalities.

E. No evidence indicates that any medication is particularly therapeutic for the dissociative process manifested by patients with DID.

200. **D.** Hypoparathyroidism can be manifested as dry skin, EPS, diarrhea, tetany, and heart failure.

A. Addison's disease (adrenal cortical insufficiency) is associated with hyperpigmentation and hypotension.

B. Cushing's syndrome (hyperadrenalism) produces symptoms of central obesity, hypertension, diabetes, and acne.

C. Hyperparathyroidism can be very similar to hypoparathyroidism in regard to psychiatric symptoms, but the physical symptoms would be different. They include weakness, anorexia, nausea, constipation, polyuria, and thirst.

E. Hyperthyroidism would likely result in warm and moist skin.

Index

Index note: page references with an *f* or a *t* indicate a figure or table on designated page; page references in **bold** indicate discussion of the subject in the Answers and Explanations section.